~

~

Pulmonary Physiology

R. David Baker

The University of Texas Medical Branch

Galveston

Alveolar air

O$_2$

0.5 μm

Aqueous layer
with surfactant

Alveolar epithelium

Capillary endothelium

Fused
basement
membranes

CO$_2$

Red cell

Blood plasma

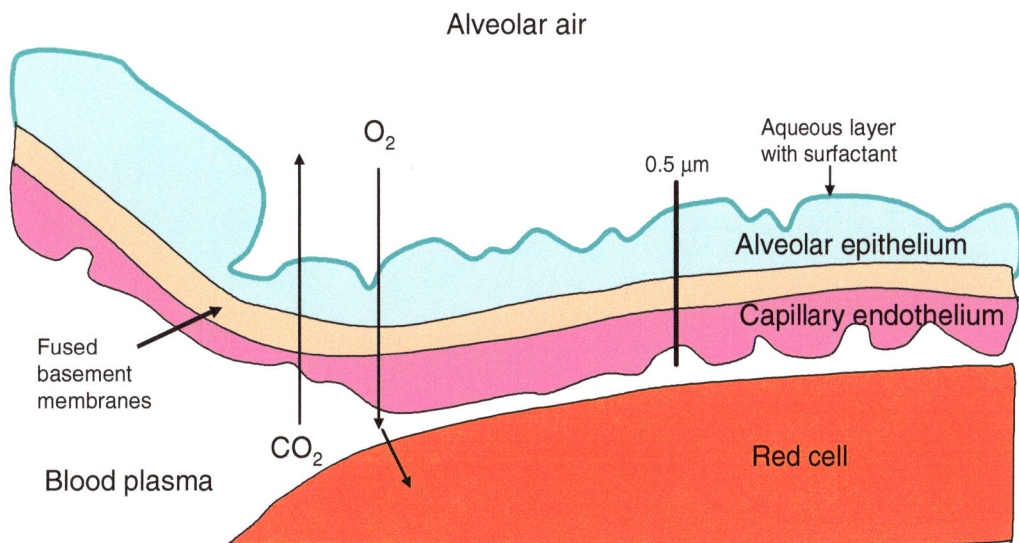

Strand
Street
Press

ISBN: 0-9741653-3-6

The drawing on the front cover is from the *Medical Illustration Library*, Sobotta Cardiology/Pulmonology Anatomy Collection, 1996, Williams & Wilkins.

Preface

This textbook is intended primarily for medical students and is meant to be a companion to my other book, <u>Cardiovascular Physiology</u>, 3rd Edition.

Many chapters contain a final section called "What Can Go Wrong?" In most cases this is just a list of problems. In some chapters these lists are accompanied by brief descriptions while in others there is not even a list. This feature is a work in progress and I invite contributions.

I am grateful to the late Dr. Malcolm Brodwick for essential encouragement. I also thank the many medical students who helped convince me to write this book. I am also indebted to Dr. Loretta Grumbles for many valuable comments and suggestions.

David Baker
May 2012

Contents

Chapter 1

Anatomy

We start this book with a very brief survey of pulmonary anatomy.

Topic 1: Whole Lungs

Figure 1
This image shows that the lungs wrap most of the way around the heart. The right lung has three main lobes and the left lung has two.

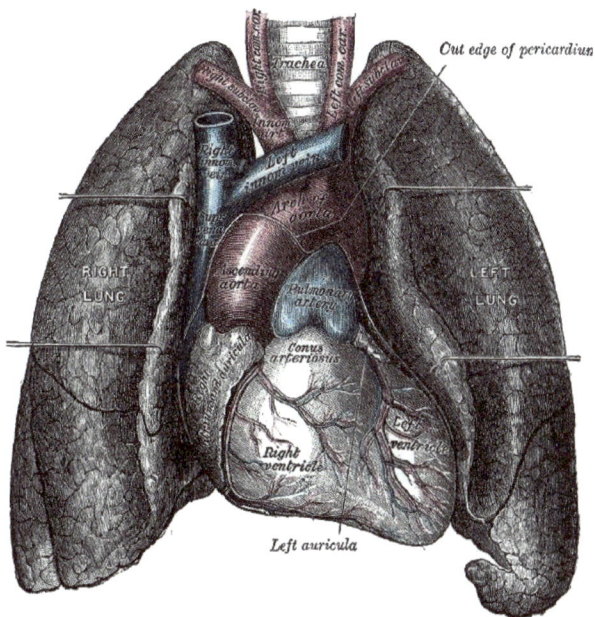

Figure 1. Drawing of lungs from the front with heart and large blood vessels for perspective. This picture is from the 1918 edition of Gray's Anatomy and is in the public domain.

Topic 2: Airways

The upper airways consist of everything from mouth and nose to the larynx. The lower airways start at the trachea followed by multiple branching into the bronchi, bronchioles, terminal bronchioles, respiratory bronchioles, alveolar ducts, and alveolar sacs. There are about 23 successive generations of branches. With each generation the branches get skinnier and shorter.

Figure 2
This image illustrates the lower airways down to roughly the third generation of bronchi. The trachea and bronchi are supported by cartilaginous rings and plates which help to prevent collapse. The bronchioles and beyond, however, have no cartilage in their walls.

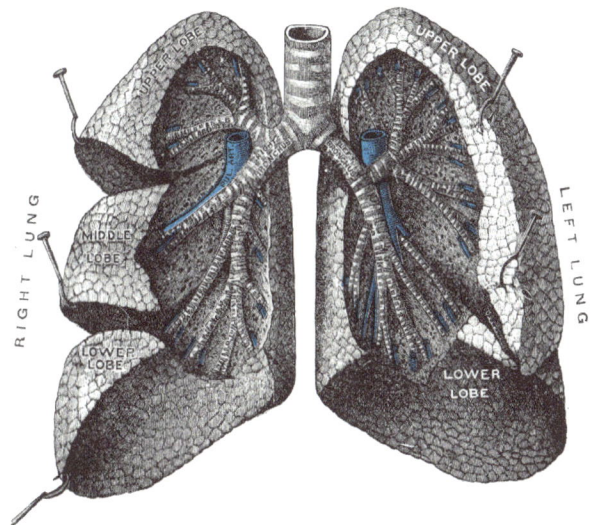

Figure 2. The lungs from the front with heart removed. The lungs are spread apart to reveal the bronchi. From the 1918 edition of Gray's Anatomy.

The following table indicates the names and approximate numbers of the successive parts in the airway system

Generation	Name	Number	Zone
0	Trachea	1	
1	Main bronchi	2	
2	Lobar bronchi	4	
3	Segmental bronchi	8	
4	Subsegmental bronchi	16	
5	Small bronchi	32	
6	Small bronchi	64	
7	Small bronchi	128	Conducting zone
8	Small bronchi	256	(no alveoli and no
9	Small bronchi	512	gas exchange)
10	Bronchioles	1024	
11	Bronchioles	2048	
12	Bronchioles	4096	
13	Bronchioles	8192	
14	Terminal bronchioles	16374	
15	Terminal bronchioles	32768	
16	Terminal bronchioles	65536	
17	Respiratory bronchioles	131072	Transitional zone
18	Respiratory bronchioles	262144	(some alveoli and
19	Respiratory bronchioles	524288	some gas exchange)
20	Alveolar ducts	$\sim 1 \times 10^6$	Respiratory zone
21	Alveolar ducts	$\sim 2 \times 10^6$	(many alveoli and
22	Alveolar ducts	$\sim 4 \times 10^6$	nearly all gas
23	Alveolar sacs	$\sim 8 \times 10^6$	exchange)
24	Alveoli	$\sim 5 \times 10^8$	

Topic 3: Alveoli   Figures 3, 4, 5, and 6

This is a section through many alveoli. A bronchiole can also be identified. The alveolar septae separating adjacent alveolar spaces are extremely thin.

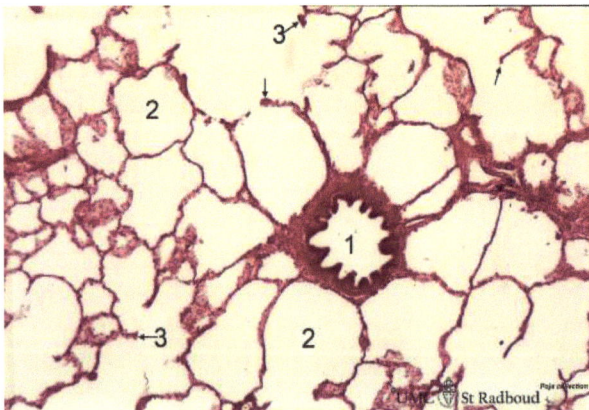

Figure 3. Section through alveoli (H & E stain). 1 = bronchiole, 2 = alveolar spaces, 3 = ? From the Poja Histology Collection – Respiratory System Subset. Downloaded from the Health Education Assets Library: Multimedia Repository.

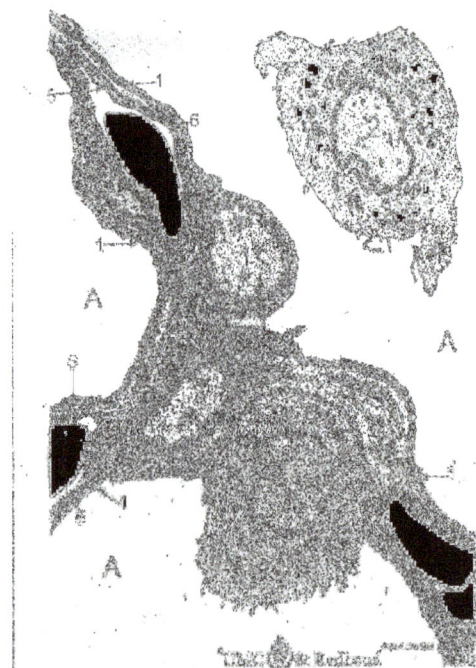

Figure 4: Transmission EM of three alveolar septae at the site where they converge. From the Poja Histology Collection – Respiratory System Subset. Downloaded from the Health Education Assets Library: Multimedia Repository.

Figure 4 shows three alveolar spaces (A) separated by alveolar septae. The three septae shown here converge at an area called a "corner". The black areas are red blood cells within capillaries.

1 is the nucleus of a type I pneumocyte whose thin cytoplasmic extensions (indicated by arrows) cover the alveolar surface
2 is a free alveolar macrophage
3 is a type II pneumocyte which secretes pulmonary surfactant.

4 is a myofibroblast.
5 indicates capillary endothelium.
6 represents the distance separating air from blood plasma, about 0.5 μm.

Figure 5 shows how the alveoli are arranged with respect to the respiratory bronchioles and alveolar ducts. This drawing does not adequately depict the extremely rich anastomosing capillary network that covers the alveoli. Figure 6 does that.

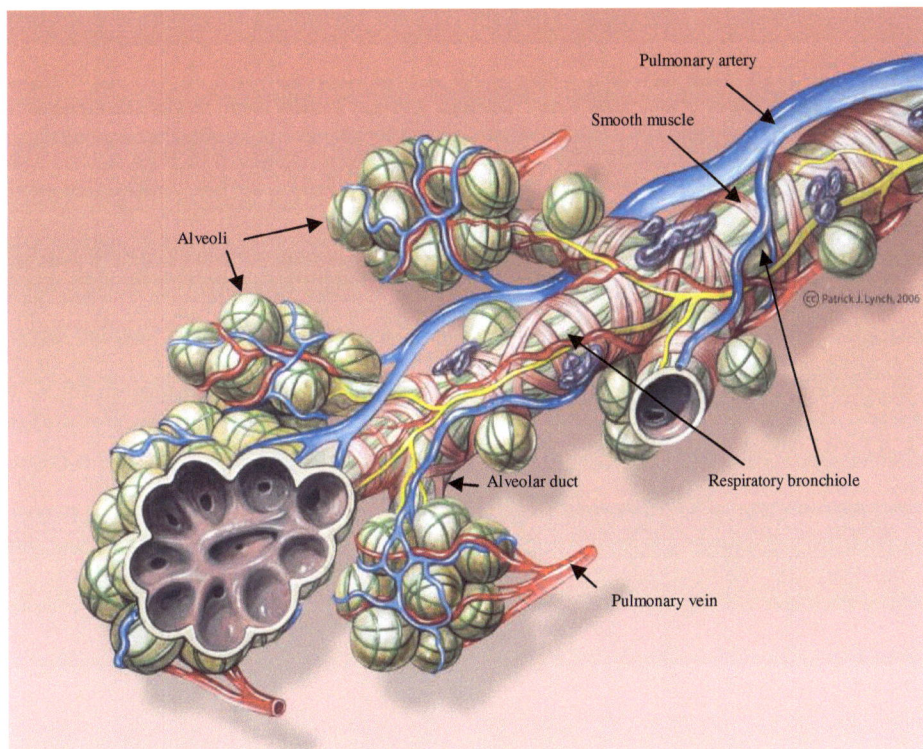

Figure 5. This drawing (minus labels) is by Patrick J. Lynch (illustrator) with C. Carl Jaffe (cardiologist), http://creativecommons.org/licenses/by/2.5. It was downloaded from Wikipedia.

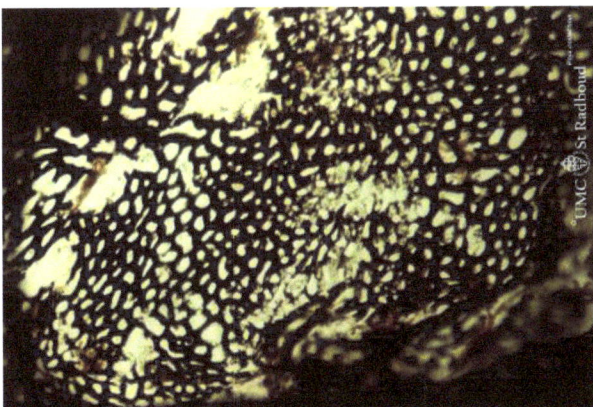

Figure 6. This image shows the dense, anastomosing capillary network covering an alveolus. The blood vessels have been filled with India ink. The larger vessels are branches of pulmonary arterioles. From the Poja Histology Collection – Respiratory System Subset. Downloaded from the Health Education Assets Library: Multimedia Repository.

Chapter 2

Breathing

Part 1: The Kinesiology of Breathing
Part 2: Lung Volumes and Capacities
Part 3: Pressures and Pressure Differences during the Breathing Cycle

Part 1: The Kinesiology of Breathing

Topic 1: Preliminaries

The lungs and all the alveoli within them are distensible; they behave as balloons that expand and compress when the thorax expands and compresses. Expansion sucks air in through the airways and compression blows air out. Changes in total lung volume exactly correspond to changes in intrathoracic volume since the outer surfaces of the lungs are stuck to the inner surfaces of the thorax by virtue of an adhesive film of fluid between the parietal and visceral pleura. This situation is similar to two microscope slides pressed together with a drop of water between them. They easily slide over each other but they cannot be pulled apart. So it is with the lungs and chest wall, they easily slide over each other but they do not normally separate.

Increased intrathoracic volume is accomplished by contraction of the muscles of inspiration. Decreased intrathoracic volume during normal quiet breathing at rest ordinarily results simply from relaxation of the muscles of inspiration, which allows elastic recoil of the lungs and chest wall. In other words, expiration is usually passive. However, during exercise and in the presence of various pulmonary diseases, expiration is active and requires the assistance of the muscles of expiration.

Normal quiet breathing at rest is called eupnea. Increased breathing during exercise is called hyperpnea.

Figure 1
The muscles of inspiration and expiration are symbolically illustrated in Figure 1.

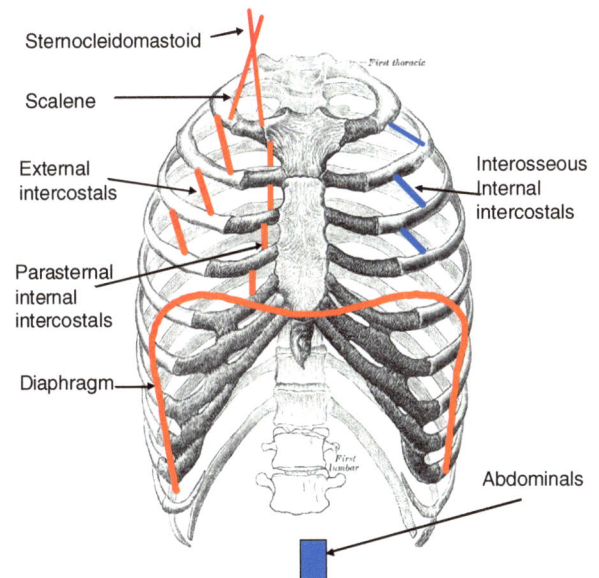

Figure 1. The muscles of inspiration and expiration: symbolic representation. Inspiration in red, expiration in blue. Rib cage is from the 1918 edition of Gray's Anatomy.

Topic 2: Inspiration

Diaphragm
The diaphragm is the main muscle of inspiration. It is a sheet of striated muscle fibers shaped like double domes. The muscle fibers arise from the lower ribs (costal part of diaphragm) and first three lumbar vertebrae (crural part of diaphragm). They converge upwards into a central tendon. As the muscle fibers of the diaphragm contract, the domes flatten toward the abdomen, increasing the longitudinal dimension of the thoracic cavity by roughly 1.5 cm during eupnea and as much as 10

cm with maximal inspiratory effort. Put a hand over your abdomen and notice that with each inspiration your hand moves outward. Contraction of the diaphragm also elevates the lower ribs.

Rhythmic trains of impulses over the phrenic nerves cause rhythmic contractions of the diaphragm. The cell bodies for the phrenics are at C4-C5, which is important for understanding breathing problems following cervical spinal cord injury.

During eupnea, contraction of the diaphragm accounts for about 2/3 of inspiration. As ventilation increases during exercise, the relative contribution of the following muscles of inspiration increases.

External Intercostals
Figure 2

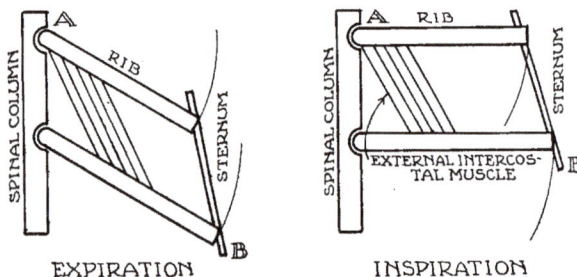

Figure 2. When the external intercostals contract, they shorten the distance between A and B, thereby moving the sternum upward and outward. From L.F. Nims, Respiration, in J.F. Fulton Ed., *A Textbook of Physiology*, 16th Ed, Saunders, 1949.

Contraction of the external intercostals expands the thoracic cavity in the lateral and anterior-posterior directions. The fibers of these muscles run from the lower edge of one rib to the upper edge of the next, sloping downward and forward. When they contract, the ribs are pulled upward and outward. Put one hand on your sternum and the other on one side of your chest. Look into a mirror and take a deep breath. Notice that both hands move upward and outward.

Motor nerves with cell bodies at thoracic levels 1 to 12 innervate the external intercostals.

Parasternal Part of Internal Intercostals
Also called interchondral part. Contraction of these muscles helps to elevate the ribs and, therefore, assists inspiration.

Scalene Muscles
The scalene muscles originate from the lower five cervical vertebrae and insert into the upper edges of the first and second ribs. Contraction of the scalene muscles elevates the first two ribs and the sternum, enlarging the rib cage, especially in its anterior-posterior dimension. The motor supply to the scalene muscles derives from the lower 5 cervical roots.

Sternocleidomastoid Muscles
The sternocleidomastoid muscles are not very active during eupnea, but are progressively recruited as ventilation increases during exercise. They are called accessory muscles of inspiration. They descend from the mastoid process and adjacent nuchal line on the skull to the front of the upper part of the manubrium sterni and the medial third of the clavicle. When they contract, the first rib and sternum are elevated, and the anterior-posterior dimension of the rib cage is increased. The motor innervation of the sternoceidomastoids derives from the spinal accessory and the second cervical nerves.

Topic 3: Expiration

Abdominal Muscles
The abdominal muscles (external oblique, internal oblique, transversus abdominis, and rectus abdominis) are the most important muscles of expiration. When they contract intra-abdominal pressure rises, which pushes the diaphragm up. In addition, they pull the lower ribs downward and inward, reducing intrathoracic volume.

Interosseous Part of Internal Intercostals
Contraction of these muscles moves the ribs downward and inward, reducing intrathoracic volume.

Topic 4: Range of Motion

Figure 3
This figure shows the range of motion of the chest wall, diaphragm, and abdominal wall during breathing.

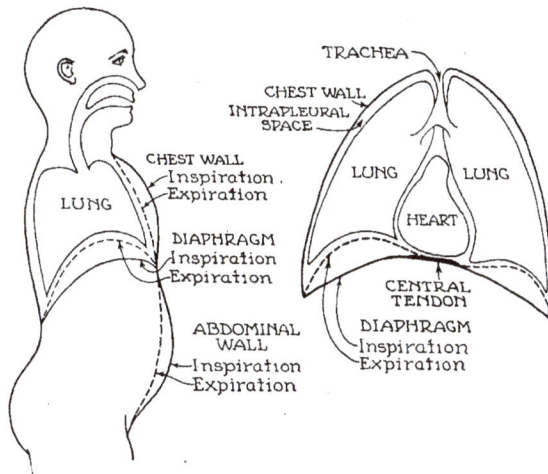

Figure 3. The drawing on the left illustrates the range of motion of the chest wall, diaphragm, and abdominal wall during maximal inspirations and expirations. The drawing on the right shows the range of motion of the diaphragm during eupnea. Note that the central part of the central tendon doesn't move much during eupnea. It can move appreciably downward during heavy breathing, pulling the heart down with it. From L.F. Nims, Respiration, in J.F. Fulton Ed., *A Textbook of Physiology*, 16th Ed, Saunders, 1949.

Part 2: Lung Volumes and Capacities

Topic 1: The Volumes

Figure 4

The total volume of air in the lungs consists of four primary volumes as shown by the left bar in Figure 4. These are the tidal volume, the inspiratory reserve volume, the expiratory reserve volume, and the residual volume. Of course, these volumes vary with body size and other factors. The values shown in Figure 4 are for a normal 70 kg adult in a sitting position.

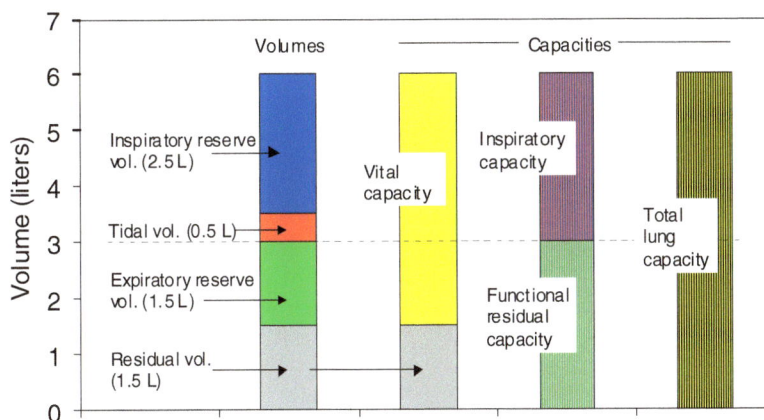

Figure 4. The primary lung volumes and capacities. Values given are for a normal 70 kg person at rest. Capacities consist of two or more of the primary lung volumes.

Tidal Volume (TV)

This is the volume of air per breath (either in or out) during regular, rhythmic breathing. At rest, our 70 kg adult has a tidal volume of about 0.5 liters/breath. Tidal volume increases during exercise.

Inspiratory Reserve Volume (IRV)

IRV is the volume of air that can be inhaled beyond a normal tidal inspiration by a maximal inspiratory effort. At rest, the IRV is about 2.5 liters in a 70 kg adult. During exercise, the increase in TV is partly at the expense of IRV; in other words, the inspiratory reserve comes into play.

Expiratory Reserve Volume (ERV)

This is the volume of air that can be exhaled beyond a normal tidal expiration by a maximal expiratory effort. At rest, the ERV is about 1.5 liters in a 70 kg adult. During exercise, this reserve also comes into play. Upon changing from a reclining to a standing posture, ERV increases appreciably at the expense of IRV. The reason for this shift is not entirely clear but has something to do with less pressure on the diaphragm from the abdominal contents.

Residual Volume (RV)

This is the volume of air that remains in the lungs after a maximal expiratory effort. No matter how hard one tries, the RV cannot be exhaled. This is largely because the more the chest wall is compressed the harder it is to compress it further while, at the same time, as the muscles of expiration actively shorten they get weaker due to the length-tension relationship. In addition, as the lungs are compressed during an intense expiratory effort small airways are also compressed, sometimes to the extent that they close altogether, trapping air in the dependent alveoli. RV is about 1.5 liters in our 70 kg person. Somewhat less than half of the RV remains in the lungs even after they are removed from the body and there is no pressure difference keeping the alveoli open. This volume is called the minimal volume (MV).

Topic 2: The Capacities

Figure 4 again
The lung capacities consist of two or more of the primary lung volumes.

Total Lung Capacity (TLC)
This is the sum of all four primary lung volumes.

Vital Capacity (VC)
Vital capacity is the volume of air that can be blown out by a maximal expiratory effort following a maximal inspiratory effort. VC is the sum of TV, IRV, and ERV. The entire VC is theoretically available for rhythmic breathing. However, under normal circumstances TV never comes close to VC, even during maximal exercise intensity – there is always unused reserve.

Inspiratory Capacity (IC)
This is the volume of air that can be sucked in by a maximal inspiratory effort following a normal tidal expiration. [IC = TV + IRV]

Functional Residual Capacity (FRC)
The FRC is the volume of air remaining in the lungs following a normal tidal expiration. The FRC is a large volume of air that considerably dilutes each inhaled tidal volume thereby reducing its O_2 concentration while increasing its CO_2 concentration. The result is that breath-by-breath fluctuations in alveolar O_2 and CO_2 concentrations are minimized. [FRC = RV + ERV]

Total Lung Capacity (again)
We have defined TLC as RV + ERV + TV + IRV. Now we see that TLC is also given by VC + RV and by IC + FRC.

Topic 3: Measurement of Lung Volumes

Measurement of lung volumes and capacities is important in clinical pulmonology and is part of standard pulmonary function testing (PFT). For example, in restrictive pulmonary diseases such as pulmonary fibrosis, lung volumes tend to be less than normal. In obstructive pulmonary diseases such as emphysema and chronic bronchitis, lung volumes are greater than normal. Spirometry can be very useful in distinguishing between these two major categories of pulmonary disease.

Spirometry
Figure 5
A spirometer is a device for measuring breathing volumes and capacities. A classic water-sealed spirometer is shown in Figure 5. There are two concentric cylinders separated by water. The inner cylinder (the bell) is partly filled with air. When the subject breathes in, the bell moves down, and a pulley arrangement causes a pen to make an upward trace on the recording paper. When the subject breaths out the bell moves up, and a downward trace is recorded.

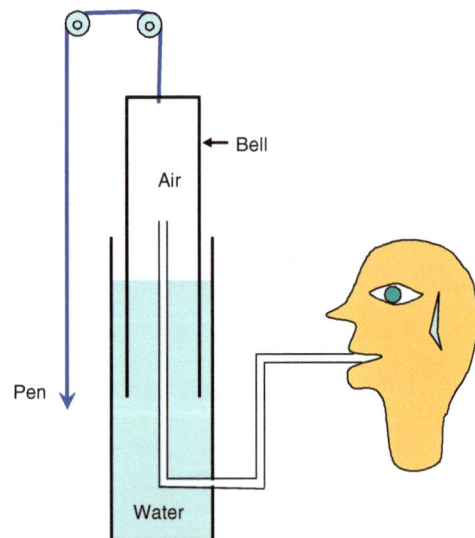

Figure 5. Diagram of classic water-sealed spirometer.

With the spirometer one can measure TV, IRV, ERV, VC, and IC as shown in Figure 6. Spirometry cannot measure RV and, therefore, cannot measure FRC and TLC.

Modern spirometers usually use a device called a pneumotachometer. A pneumotach directly measures the velocity of airflow and then calculates the rate of airflow by integrating over time. Pneumotachometers still can't determine RV since by definition it can't be exhaled.

Figure 6
Here is the kind of trace that can be obtained from spirometry. This figure might be useful for reference.

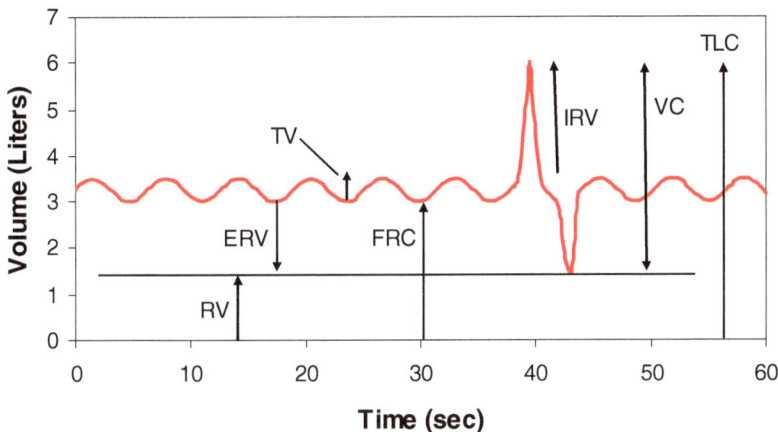

Figure 6. Spirogram.

RV = residual volume
ERV = expiratory reserve volume
TV = tidal volume
FRC = functional residual capacity
IRV = inspiratory reserve volume
VC = vital capacity
TLC = total lung capacity

Note: The eupneic tidal volume trace was generated from the equation for a sine wave, which is not really accurate.

Measurement of RV, FRC, and TLC
There are three standard methods for measuring RV, FRC, and TLC. The first two are not used much anymore, but they are presented here for completeness.

The Helium Dilution Method
The air in the bell of a spirometer is diluted with about 10% helium. The subject breathes into and out of the spirometer. It is assumed that no helium enters the blood from the lungs. If this is true, then the spirometer together with lungs and airways is a closed system through which the helium gradually equilibrates. As it equilibrates, the helium concentration decreases in the spirometer and increases in the lungs until finally it is the same concentration everywhere. The original amount of

helium in the spirometer is known and there was no helium originally in the lungs. The final concentration of helium in the spirometer allows calculation of the total volume in which it is distributed. After subtracting the gas volume in the spirometer and in the tubes leading to and from the subject, lung volume can be calculated. If the procedure is stopped at FRC, then the lung volume calculated is the FRC. RV can then be calculated by subtracting ERV.

The usual justification given in textbooks for the assumption that helium does not enter the blood in appreciable amounts is that it is essentially insoluble in blood, which is not true. Helium has about 1/3 the solubility that oxygen has in blood. However, the error incurred by helium diffusion into blood is very small and can be ignored.

The Nitrogen Washout Method
The subject breathes in 100% oxygen and breaths out into a spirometer that initially contains no nitrogen. One-way valves in the system direct the flows. Gradually all the nitrogen that was originally in the lungs is exhaled into the spirometer. When no more nitrogen can be detected in the outflow tube (using a nitrogen analyzer), the procedure is stopped and the total amount of nitrogen exhaled is measured. This is assumed to equal the total volume of nitrogen in the lungs at the beginning of the procedure. From this value and the fact that initially the air in the lungs was about 80% nitrogen, the initial volume of air in the lungs can be calculated. If the procedure was started at FRC, the lung volume calculated is the FRC.

The nitrogen washout technique assumes that all the nitrogen collected was initially in the lungs and airways and that no appreciable amount of nitrogen enters the lungs from the blood during the procedure. This assumption cannot be strictly true since nitrogen is about as diffusible as oxygen, but again, the error is probably not large.

The Body Plethysmograph Method
The body plethysmograph is an airtight box in which the subject sits and breaths normally for awhile through the mouthpiece and associated tubing to and from the outside room. The subject

has a clip on the nose to prevent nose breathing. Just at the end of a normal expiration (*i.e.* at FRC) the operator remotely closes a shutter in the breathing tube so that no air can be inhaled. The next inspiratory effort causes the lungs to expand and since no air can enter, the pressure drops according to Boyle's Law. [In case you have forgotten, Boyle's Law states that in a closed chamber containing an ideal gas at constant temperature, the product of pressure and volume is constant, so as volume goes up pressure goes down.] Airway pressure at the end of the inspiratory effort is measured by a pressure transducer connected to the breathing tube.

Now if we could determine how much the lungs expanded during this inspiratory effort we could calculate the FRC using Boyle's Law. This is where the box comes in. During the inspiratory effort, the air pressure in the box increases slightly due to the expansion of the thorax. A sensitive pressure transducer in the box measures this increase. The amount of thoracic expansion can be calculated by Boyle's Law, but it is more accurate to use a previously determined calibration curve obtained by injecting known volumes of air into the box with the subject inside. Of course, all the calculations are done automatically by computer. The basic equation for FRC derived from Boyle's Law is

$$FRC = \frac{P_{final} \times \Delta V}{P_{initial} - P_{final}}$$

ΔV is determined by the pressure change in the previously calibrated box. You could probably derive this equation yourself from the following starting point: $P_{initial} \times FRC = P_{final} \times V_{final}$, but, on the other hand, why bother? Also, don't bother memorizing these equations.

The helium dilution and nitrogen washout methods underestimate FRC whenever there is air trapped in unventilated alveoli. Significant air trapping can occur in various pulmonary diseases, *e.g.* emphysema, and this error can be quite large. Thus, the body plethysmograph method is preferred. A large discrepancy between FRC measured by body plethysmography and FRC measured by helium dilution or nitrogen washout can be diagnostic of air trapping.

Part 3: Pressures and Pressure Differences during the Breathing Cycle

The values for pressures are always given with respect to atmospheric pressure. For example, if intrapleural pressure is 755 mmHg while atmospheric pressure is 760 mmHg, intrapleural pressure is said to be -5 mmHg. This same convention is used for blood pressures. Pressures can be expressed in mmHg. Many pulmonary physiologists and clinicians prefer cm of H_2O. Both units are used below. Pressure expressed in mmHg is about ¾ of the pressure expressed in cm H_2O.

There are four pressures and five pressure differences that are important in breathing.

Topic 1: The Pressures   Figure 7

Pressure at Airway Opening (P$_{AO}$)
This is the air pressure at the mouth or nose (or sometimes endotracheal catheter). Ordinarily P_{AO} equals atmospheric pressure (*i.e.* is zero), but not necessarily during mechanical ventilation.

Pressure at Body Surface (P$_{BS}$)
This is the air pressure just outside the chest wall. P_{BS} ordinarily equals atmospheric pressure and P_{AO}, but not necessarily during mechanical ventilation or water immersion.

Alveolar Pressure (P$_A$)
This is the air pressure in the alveoli (compared, as always, to atmospheric pressure). P_A is also called intrapulmonary pressure. Actual measurement of P_A requires use of the body plethysmograph as described later.

Intrapleural Pressure (P$_{PL}$)
This is the force per unit of surface area that tries to pull the visceral and parietal pleura apart. This force is caused partly by the continuous tendency of the lungs to recoil to a smaller volume (due to passive elasticity and surface tension). It is also caused by the tendency of the chest wall to expand, partly by passive elastic recoil and partly, during inspiration, by active contraction of the muscles of inspiration. During spontaneous eupnea, P_{PL} ranges

from about -4 mmHg at end-expiration to about -7 mmHg at end-inspiration. It cannot be measured directly by a pressure transducer unless an air space (pneumothorax) is artificially created between the pleura. Ordinarily, P_{PL} is measured by measuring the pressure in the thoracic part of the esophagus. This is possible since baseline pressure in the thoracic esophagus essentially equals P_{PL}. Esophageal pressure is determined using a tube inserted *via* the nose and pharynx. This tube often has a balloon on its tip, but it can be just an open tipped catheter. In either case, the other end is connected to a pressure transducer outside the body.

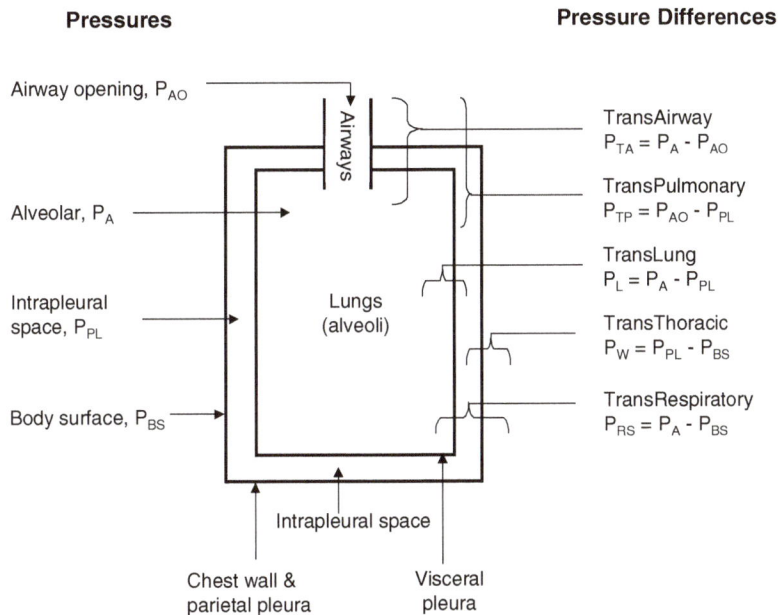

Pressures   **Pressure Differences**

TransAirway
$P_{TA} = P_A - P_{AO}$

TransPulmonary
$P_{TP} = P_{AO} - P_{PL}$

TransLung
$P_L = P_A - P_{PL}$

TransThoracic
$P_W = P_{PL} - P_{BS}$

TransRespiratory
$P_{RS} = P_A - P_{BS}$

Figure 7. Breathing pressures and pressure differences.

Two additional pressures should be mentioned here: maximum inspiratory pressure (MIP) and maximum expiratory pressure (MEP). These pressures are measured in pulmonary function labs to test respiratory muscle strength. The patient, with nose clipped and mouth tightly sealed around a tube, applies full inspiratory or expiratory strength against a pressure transducer. MIP is measured during a maximal inspiratory effort at residual volume (RV) since the inspiratory muscles are strongest when they are longest. MEP is measured during maximal expiratory effort at total lung capacity (TLC) for the same reason.

TransAirway, P_{TA}
The transairway pressure difference is defined as $P_A - P_{AO}$. This pressure drop occurs through the airways as air is sucked in or blown out. Resistance to airflow along the airways causes it. When the airways are open but there is no airflow, for example at end-inspiration or end-expiration, P_{TA} is zero. Airway resistance will be discussed later.

TransPulmonary, P_{TP}
The transpulmonary pressure difference is defined as $P_{AO} - P_{PL}$. During spontaneous eupnea, P_{TP} is always positive. During inspiration, P_{TP} expands the lungs. This reduces P_A and, consequently air is sucked in, overcoming the elastic resistance of the lungs and the flow resistance of the airways. During expiration, P_{TP} becomes less positive, allowing the lungs to recoil against flow resistance in the airways.

TransLung, P_L
The translung pressure difference is defined as $P_A - P_{PL}$. This pressure difference keeps the alveoli inflated. When airflow is zero, P_L is the same as P_{TP}, since in this case there is no pressure drop through the airways and $P_A = P_{AO}$. P_L is sometimes called the elastic recoil pressure of the lungs, since it is a measure of how forcefully the lungs try to retract elastically away from the chest wall.

TransThoracic, P_W
The transthoracic pressure difference is defined as $P_{PL} - P_{BS}$. Just as P_L is a measure of the inward elastic recoil of the lungs, P_W is a measure of the outward elastic recoil of the chest wall. P_W is also called the trans-chest-wall pressure difference, which accounts for the W in the symbol. As long as P_{BS} is zero, P_W is the same as P_{PL}. Notice that P_W is equal and opposite to P_{TP} as long as $P_{AO} = P_{BS}$. P_W is also equal and opposite to P_L when no air is flowing. In other words, under static conditions the lungs are trying to pull the chest wall inward with the same force that the chest wall is trying to expand the lungs.

TransRespiratory, P_{RS}

The transrespiratory pressure difference is defined as P_A - P_{BS}. The RS in the symbol is for respiratory system. P_{RS} is a measure of <u>net</u> elastic recoil – lungs and chest wall together. Notice that when P_{AO} = P_{BS} (the usual situation), P_{RS} = P_{TA}. In fact, the terms transrespiratory pressure difference and transairway pressure difference are sometimes used synonymously.

Warning: Some authors do not distinguish between P_{TP} and P_L, and define them both as P_A - P_{PL}. I think this is a mistake, and it can certainly be confusing.

Perhaps many of you have noticed that around this point in pulmonary physiology remembering the symbols becomes a challenge. Frequent reference to Figure 7 might help. In addition, the final page of this chapter summarizes all the symbols used here.

Topic 3: The Breathing Cycle

Figure 8

As the inspiratory muscles expand the thorax during inspiration, intrapleural pressure (P_{PL}) decreases. If there were no resistance to flow in the airways, it would decrease less (dashed line). As P_{PL} decreases, the lungs are expanded thereby decreasing alveolar pressure (P_A) and sucking air in from the outside through the airways. As air continues to come in, P_A gradually increases, until it finally reaches zero at the end of inspiration and airflow stops for an instant. Now, as the inspiratory muscles relax, P_{PL} rises and eventually reaches its end-expiratory value. If there were no resistance to flow, it would rise less steeply (dashed line). P_A

rises at first during expiration and then falls back to zero. Toward the end of expiration, nothing much happens. Once P_A reaches zero there is no more airflow. This short period of no airflow that precedes the next inspiration is called the expiratory pause.

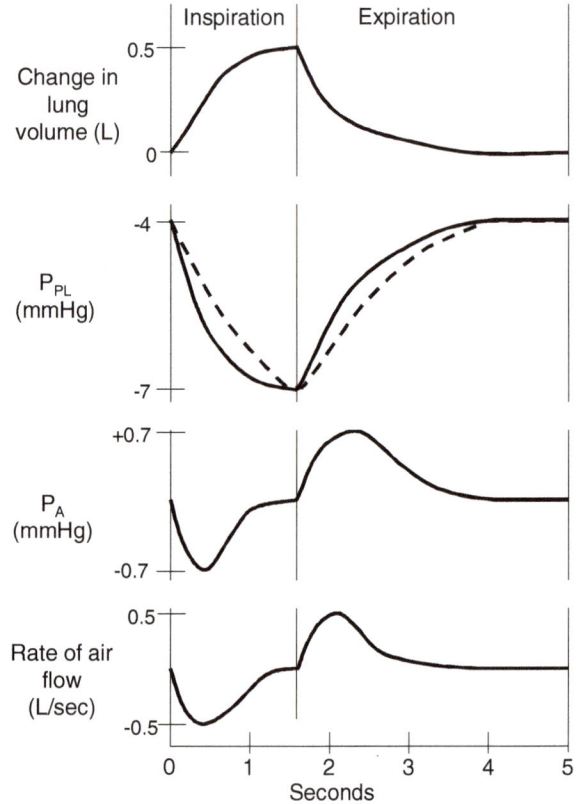

Figure 8. Pressures, flows, and volume changes during a normal breathing cycle at rest.

Part 4: Symbols Used in this Chapter

Symbol	Name	Definitions	Synonym
Lung Volumes			
TV	Tidal volume		
IRV	Inspiratory reserve volume		
ERV	Expiratory reserve volume		
RV	Residual volume		
MV	Minimal volume		
Lung Capacities			
TLC	Total lung capacity	TV + IRV + ERV + RV	
VC	Vital capacity	TV + IRV + ERV	
IC	Inspiratory capacity	TV + IRV	
FRC	Functional residual capacity	ERV + RS	
Pressures			
P_{AO}	Airway opening pressure		
P_{BS}	Body surface pressure		
P_A	Alveolar pressure		Intrapulmonary
P_{PL}	Intrapleural pressure		
MIP	Maximum inspiratory p		
MEP	Maximum expiratory p		
Pressure Differences			
P_{TA}	Transairway	$P_A - P_{AO}$	Transrespiratory
P_{TP}	Transpulmonary	$P_{AO} - P_{PL}$	
P_L	Translung	$P_A - P_{PL}$	Elastic recoil of lungs
P_W	Transthoracic	$P_{PL} - P_{BS}$	Trans-chest-wall
P_{RS}	Transrespiratory	$P_A - P_{BS}$	Transairway
Miscellaneous			
R_{AW}	Airway resistance	$(P_A - P_{AO})/\dot{V}$	
$\dot{V}$	Rate of air flow		
EPP	Equal pressure point		
PFT	Pulmonary function tests		

Chapter 3

Pulmonary Mechanics

Part 1: Static Pressure-Volume Relations for the Lungs

Topic 1: Static Compliance of the Lungs

Figure 1

Here we plot total volume of air in the lungs as a function of the transmural pressure difference across the alveolar wall, *i.e.* the translung pressure difference (P_L). The big loop is for the vital capacity; the small loop is for a tidal volume during eupnea. In each case, there are two curves, one for inspiration, and one for expiration. The slope at any point along any of these curves is called lung compliance. Compliance is a measure of the ease with which a hollow compartment can be inflated or deflated by a small change in transmural pressure. Compliance depends on the distensibility of the tissue (alveolar walls, *etc.*) and on the capacity of the organ. For example, both lungs in parallel have twice the compliance of a single lung. Often, for comparison among people of different sizes, compliance is divided by FRC – this is called specific compliance.

The compliance curves shown in Figure 1 are obtained by having the subject breath in or out incrementally with pauses. During the pauses, no air moves but the airways are kept open. Volume changes are measured with a spirometer, and intrapleural pressure (P_{PL}) is measured from the esophagus. The curves in Figure 1 are called static compliance curves because no air is moving at the time pressure and volume measurements are made. As long as no air is moving $P_{AO} = P_A$ and $P_L = P_{TP} = -P_{PL}$.

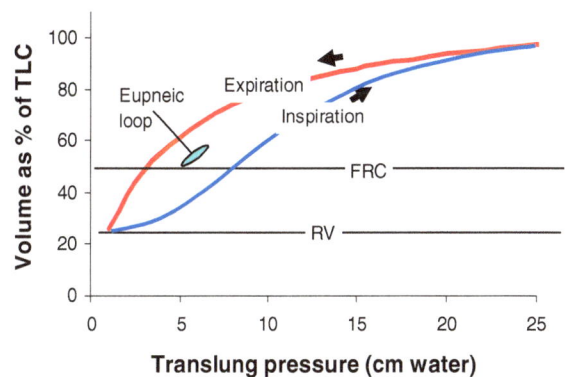

Figure 1. Static inspiratory and expiratory compliance curves for the lungs. The big loop represents the data for the vital capacity (*i.e.* from RV to TLC). The small loop is for a normal tidal volume.

Similar static compliance curves can be obtained using excised lungs from experimental animals. P_L can be changed either by increasing P_A (as in positive pressure breathing) or by decreasing outside pressure (as in normal breathing). When there is no distending pressure (*i.e.* $P_L = 0$) the lung volume is called minimal volume.

The deflation curve is not simply a retrace of the inflation curve. This phenomenon is called hysteresis. Let's first look at the inflation curve.

Inflation Curve

At very low lung volumes inflation is difficult; a little inflation requires a lot of pressure change. Low inflationary compliance near RV is thought to owe mainly to the fact that near RV many alveoli and perhaps small bronchioles are completely collapsed and it takes more transmural pressure to open collapsed alveoli than it does to expand open alveoli. The explanation for this behavior is complex and we don't need it. A similar phenomenon occurs when you try to inflate a rubber balloon – hard at first, but then it gets easier.

Also, notice that at very high lung volumes (near total lung capacity, TLC) inflation is difficult. Reduced inflationary compliance at high lung volumes results from two factors: 1) increased resistance to stretch of collagen and elastin fiber networks as these fiber networks expand, and 2) increased alveolar surface tension due to dilution of alveolar surfactant (to be discussed below).

Deflation Curve
At high lung volumes, incremental decreases in transmural pressure have relatively small effects on lung volume. I have found no satisfactory explanation for this fact. At low lung volumes, the deflationary curve is steep, probably because it is easy to collapse alveoli at low distending pressures.

Static Compliance Curve over Normal Volume Range during Eupnea
A normal tidal volume in a 70 kg person at rest is roughly 500 ml. Over this range, as shown in Figure 1, there is not much hysteresis and we can usually assume that the pressure-volume relationship is simply a straight line. This assumption will be used later when we compare the dynamic pressure-volume relationship to the static pressure-volume relationship.

Effects of Diseases on Lung Compliance
Figure 2
Static lung compliance is reduced in pulmonary fibrosis, congestive heart failure, and pneumonia. It is increased in emphysema and, to some extent, during normal aging. Figure 2 shows some examples. Only deflationary compliance curves are drawn. Notice that in emphysema, an obstructive disorder that involves breakdown of pulmonary elastic fibers, the volumes at any P_L are large; this includes residual volume. In pulmonary fibrosis, the volumes are low.

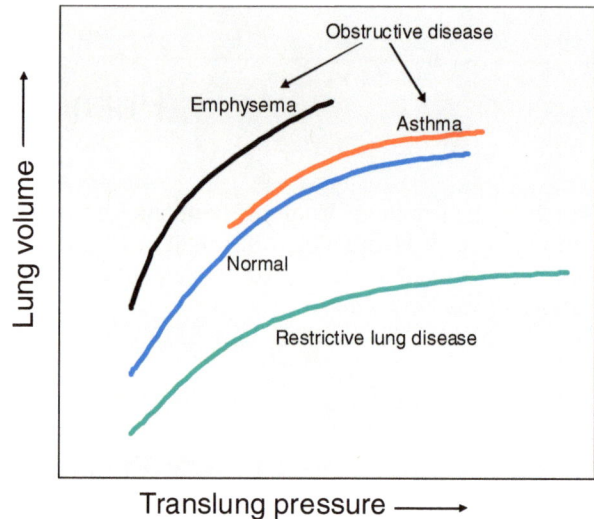

Figure 2. Effects of various pulmonary diseases on expiratory pressure-volume curves for the lungs. In each case, the lowest volume is residual volume and the highest volume is total lung capacity.

Topic 2: Recoil Tendency of the Lungs

Throughout the entire vital capacity, the lungs are constantly trying to recoil to a smaller volume. The only reason they don't is that the chest wall won't let them. If trauma or surgery results in a large opening between the intrapleural space and the outside, the lungs collapse to their minimal volume. What are the forces responsible for the recoil tendency of the lungs? There are two: tissue elasticity and alveolar surface tension.

Tissue Elasticity
A network of collagen and elastin fibers courses through all of the interstitial space of the lungs. The individual collagen and elastin fibers are highly elastic; *i.e.* they resist being stretched. They develop passive tension when stretched which tries to pull them back to their slack length, just like a rubber band. In addition, the fibrous network resists being distorted and tries to spring back to its slack configuration, much like a nylon stocking.

Alveolar Surface Tension
What is Alveolar Surface Tension?
A thin film of water covers the alveolar surface and makes contact with alveolar air, creating an air-water interface. At any air-water interface, there is considerable surface tension in the water. You have probably all been successful at one time or another at floating a pin or paper clip on the surface of water. The pin doesn't sink unless the surface film

is broken. The surface film is really just water molecules that are attracted to each other asymmetrically. In bulk water, every water molecule is attracted to other water molecules in all directions. The attractive forces are rather strong, but since they are in all directions there is no net force on any one molecule. The situation is different at the surface where water molecules are not attracted much by the overlying air molecules. This asymmetric pull on the surface molecules has the effect of pulling them together quite strongly. They resist being pulled apart. The result is that an air-water interface is constantly trying to get smaller. Drops of water or soap bubbles tend to assume a spherical shape because a sphere has the smallest possible surface area for any given volume. The force per unit distance along the surface required to expand an air-water interface is called the surface tension. It is also called interfacial tension.

Is Alveolar Surface Tension Important?
Yes. Alveolar surface tension contributes roughly 2/3 of the total recoil tendency of the lungs.

Figure 3
In 1929, von Neergaard performed a simple experiment. He inflated isolated cat lungs with either air or saline. Saline was used for getting rid of the air-water interface. Figure 3 shows that the static compliance of saline-inflated lungs is far greater than that of air-inflated lungs. Saline also eliminates most of the hysteresis; the conclusion from this observation is that surfactant is responsible for the hysteresis, but the mechanism is not entirely clear.

Pulmonary Surfactant
Alveolar surface tension would be much higher and we would not be able to breath if it were not for the presence of a detergent called pulmonary surfactant. Detergents reduce interfacial tension. If you drop just a tiny amount of detergent into the water on which your paper clip is floating, it immediately sinks. Detergents reduce interfacial tension by interposing themselves at the surface between some of the water molecules. The attraction between detergent molecules and water molecules is far less than that between water and water; so overall, the surface "film" tends to retract less forcefully. [Incidentally, one of the main ways that detergents help clean your skin and dishes is by reduction of interfacial tension between fat globs and water

allowing the fat globs to be broken down to smaller droplets having a much larger total surface area.]

Experimentally, most of the pulmonary surfactant can be washed out of the lungs with saline. Compliance, determined during air filling, decreases enormously. Without pulmonary surfactant, lung recoil would be so powerful that inspiration would be practically impossible. This is, in fact, the situation in some premature infants since pulmonary surfactant is not secreted in adequate amounts nor does it reach its most effective composition until rather late during gestation. The condition is called infant respiratory distress syndrome. It can be treated by instilling synthetic surfactant into the lungs.

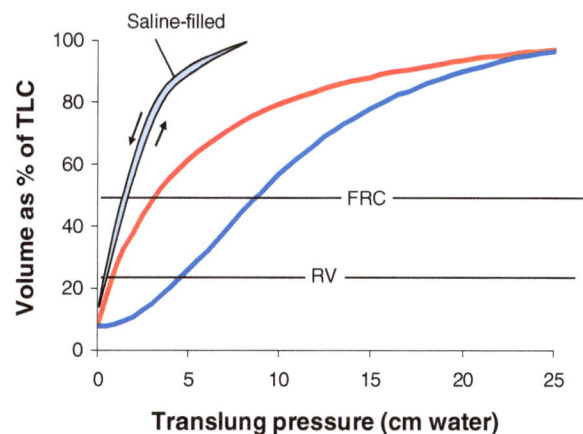

Figure 3. Effect of eliminating the air-water interface in the lungs on static lung compliance. Cat data scaled up to human size.

Pulmonary surfactant is secreted by type II alveolar epithelial cells by exocytosis of lamellar bodies. These cells generate surfactant molecules by synthesizing them from fatty acids. Some of the fatty acids are captured from blood. If anything happens to compromise blood supply to a portion of lung, such as a pulmonary embolus, surfactant secretion in the affected region can become insufficient.

There is a rapid turnover of pulmonary surfactant. Alveolar macrophages continuously gobble up some of it. Some is absorbed across the alveolar epithelium and carried away in lymph, some is absorbed back into type II cells, and some migrates into small bronchioles and is carried up the mucociliary escalator (see Chapter 13, p.115). Thus, the type II cells must continuously synthesize and secrete new surfactant.

Composition and Properties of Pulmonary Surfactant

Pulmonary surfactant consists of a mixture of phospholipids and proteins. The most abundant phospholipid is dipalmitoyl phosphatidylcholine. This is lecithin whose acyl chains are both made of palmitic acid. Other phospholipids in pulmonary surfactant include phosphatidylglycerol and phosphatidylcholines that have unsaturated fatty acid chains rather then palmitic acid. Phospholipids are nearly insoluble in water, unlike certain other detergents like soap. But one end of a phospholipid molecule can dissolve in water. In the case of lecithin, the water-soluble part is the glycerylcholine moiety. The acyl chains can dissolve in fats or fat solvents. This kind of molecule is called an amphiphile, meaning that one end loves water and the other loves fat. The end that loves fat is also reasonably compatible with air. If you put some lecithin in a beaker containing water, most of it just sinks as lumps. But some of the molecules migrate (by diffusion or convection) to the air-water interface where they intersperse between the surface water molecules, reducing the air-water interfacial tension. The acyl chains stick out into the air and the water soluble parts remain in the water.

There are also proteins in the exocytotic secretion from alveolar type II epithelial cells. The proteins constitute about 10% of the total secretion, and about half of this is plasma protein, mainly albumin. In addition, there are four special proteins: SP-A, SP-B, SP-C, and SP-D. SP stands for surfactant protein. Two of these are involved in immune responses (SP-A and SP-D). The others (SP-B, SP-C, and perhaps albumin) are involved in assisting the entry of the phospholipids into the air-water interface. There is a hereditary disease in which SP-B is absent. This condition is fatal in newborns unless lung transplantation is provided.

Pulmonary Surfactant and Alveolar Surface Area

Consider an alveolar air-water interface. The interface has a certain number of phospholipid molecules interspersed among the water molecules. These phospholipid molecules reduce the surface tension. Now, if the alveoli are inflated, the surface area of the air-water interface increases and the phospholipid molecules in the interface are diluted. As they are diluted, they reduce the interfacial tension less and less. Thus, as alveoli are inflated during inspiration, they become harder to inflate

further because of increased surface tension. As they deflate during expiration, the interfacial concentration of surfactant increases and interfacial tension progressively decreases. Thus, due to both surface tension changes and tissue elasticity changes, lung recoil tendency increases with inspiration and decreases with expiration.

Topic 3: Alveolar Stability

Alveoli exist in a wide range of sizes. If the tension in the walls (including both tissue elastic tension and surface tension) is the same for all sizes of alveoli, it might be expected that the small alveoli would all empty into the larger alveoli. This expectation derives from the Laplace equation, which for a sphere is:

$$P = \frac{2T}{r}$$

where P is pressure, T is total wall tension, and r is radius.

Small alveoli should have higher pressures than larger alveoli since their radii are smaller. Since all alveoli are interconnected by the airway system, the air in those with higher pressures should flow into those with lower pressures. Most of the alveoli then would collapse (atelectasis). This phenomenon can easily be demonstrated using interconnected soap bubbles of different sizes – the small ones empty into the large ones.

In fact, it is reasonable to expect that tissue tension plus surface tension is nearly the same for all alveoli, so how is it possible to maintain a stable situation with small alveoli connected to large alveoli? The answer is that individual alveoli are not free like individual soap bubbles are. They are held in a meshwork of interstitial tissue and other alveoli. Any single alveolus cannot collapse without pulling on its neighbors, or expand without pushing on its neighbors. In other words, they exist in an interdependent meshwork, and the elastic forces that exist in this meshwork override any tendency for instability that might be caused by surface tension problems. This phenomenon is called the principle of alveolar interdependence. The success of alveolar interdependence in maintaining alveolar stability is greatly facilitated by pulmonary surfactant. If surface tension at the alveolar air-water interface were not greatly reduced by pulmonary surfactant, small alveoli would empty into the larger ones in spite of alveolar interdependence. In fact, any situation that results in a deficiency of pulmonary surfactant can lead to extensive atelectasis.

Part 2: Static Pressure-Volume Relations for the Chest Wall and for the Chest Wall and Lungs Combined

Topic 1: Static Compliance Curve for the Whole System

Figure 4

In experimental animals, the static compliance curve for the chest wall can be determined after removing the lungs from the chest. But in people, a more satisfactory approach is to determine the pressure-volume relationship for the whole system (chest wall with intact lungs inside) and then, together with the pressure-volume relationship for the lungs, calculate the curve for the chest wall.

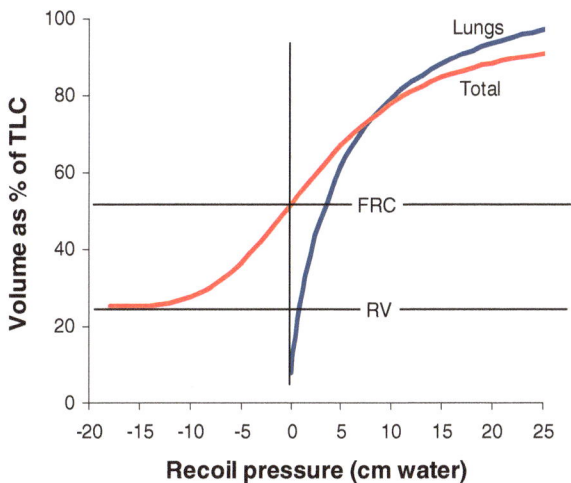

Figure 4. Static compliance curve for the whole system (chest wall + lungs) compared to that of the lungs alone (expiration only). Both of these curves can be directly obtained on people (except the part of the lung curve below RV).

Static compliance of the whole system can be determined from measurements of volume changes and P_{RS} during positive pressure or negative pressure mechanical ventilation with completely relaxed respiratory muscles. Such a relationship is shown in Figure 4. Static compliance of the lungs can be determined as described above from measurements of P_{PL}. Customarily, only the expiratory compliance curves are used for this kind of analysis.

Topic 3: Static Compliance Curve for the Chest Wall

The lungs and chest wall consist of two elastances in series (elastance is the reciprocal of compliance). Elastances in series sum. Therefore,

$$\frac{1}{Total\ C} = \frac{1}{Lung\ C} + \frac{1}{Chest\ wall\ C}$$

C = compliance

Figure 5

Having determined the total compliance curve and the lung compliance curve, we can solve for chest wall compliance at any volume and then construct the chest wall compliance curve. All three curves are plotted in Figure 5.

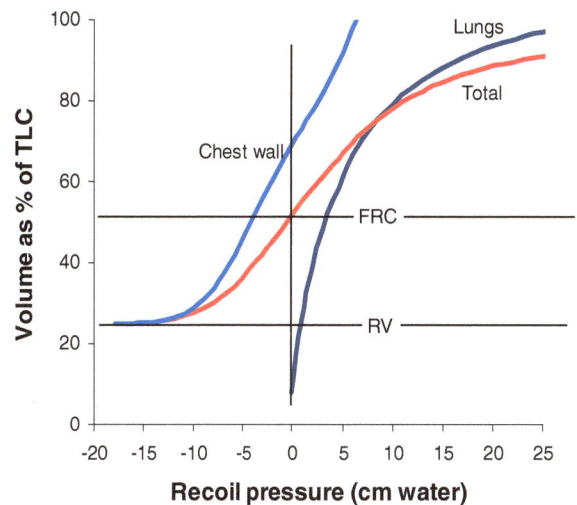

Figure 5. The three compliance curves. Recoil pressure is P_{RS} (transrespiratory) for whole system, P_L (translung) for lungs, and P_W (transthoracic) for chest wall.

This plot can be confusing since recoil pressure (the abscissa) is different for each of the three curves. For the lungs, recoil pressure is P_L. For the chest wall, recoil pressure is P_W. For the lungs and chest wall combined, recoil pressure is P_{RS}. Negative recoil pressures mean that the structure involved (chest wall or whole system) is trying passively to recoil outward. Positive recoil pressures mean that the structure involved (lung, chest wall, or whole system) is trying passively to recoil inward.

There are some important observations to be made from Figure 5.

- All the way from residual volume to about 70% of total lung capacity, negative P_W is required to keep the chest wall from passively expanding. This means that in this entire volume range the chest wall is constantly trying to recoil to a larger volume, working against the tendency of the lungs to recoil to a smaller volume. Only after the thorax is inflated to more than about 70% of normal TLC does it actually resist further inflation.
- When lung elastic recoil is equal and opposite to chest wall elastic recoil, P_{RS} is zero, and the volume of the system is at FRC. In other words, FRC is the resting volume of the system; movement away from FRC in either direction requires contraction of respiratory muscles.
- The curve for the whole system shows the P_{RS} that must be achieved by the respiratory muscles, or by a mechanical ventilator, in order to move a given volume of air.
- When lung volume is about 70% of total lung capacity, the chest wall itself is at its equilibrium position – it is not trying to recoil in either direction. At smaller lung volumes, the chest wall is trying to recoil outward and at greater lung volumes, it is trying to recoil inward. At all volumes, the lungs are trying to recoil inward.

- If P_L and P_W both become zero, as they would if the chest wall were widely opened to the outside by trauma or surgery, the chest wall passively expands to about 70% of normal TLC, and the lungs passively recoil to their minimal volume, which is less than half of residual volume. This condition is called an open pneumothorax.

Chest wall compliance is reduced in obesity, fibrothorax, kyphoscoliosis, and aging.

Topic 4: Relaxation Pressure-Volume Curves

There is a technique that can generate static pressure-volume curves for the lungs, chest wall, and whole respiratory system all at once. The subject, with nose clipped, inhales or exhales a known volume (determined by a spirometer) and then the external airway is shut off and the subject completely relaxes all muscles of respiration. Airway pressure and intrapleural pressure (esophagus) are measured. Translung pressure is given by airway pressure minus intrapleural pressure. Transthoracic pressure is given by intrapleural pressure. Transrespiratory pressure is given by airway pressure. These transmural pressures are the recoil pressures. The procedure is repeated throughout the entire possible range of lung volumes. Results similar to those shown in Figure 5 are obtained, but the technique is difficult and requires very well-trained subjects.

Part 3: Dynamic Pressure-Volume Relations

Topic 1: Dynamic Pressure-Volume Loop

Recall Figure 8 in Chapter 2. There it was shown that during a normal inspiration intrapleural pressure drops lower than it would if no air were moving, and during expiration intrapleural pressure rises higher than it would if no air were moving. Also recall that during inspiration alveolar pressure decreases, and during expiration it increases. These changes are necessary for sucking air in and blowing air out.

Intrapleural pressure must change more than it does in a static experiment because when air is flowing there is viscous resistance through the airways and there is frictional resistance related to thoracic tissues moving over each other. Intrapleural pressure must change enough during inspiration to overcome airway resistance and tissue resistance, in addition to overcoming elastic recoil of the lungs.

For perspective, during normal eupneic breathing the change in intrapleural pressure required to overcome elastic recoil of the lungs is about 3 or 4 times larger than that required for overcoming airway and tissue resistances combined. Tissue resistance is only about 25% of airway resistance.

Figure 6
Figure 6 shows a pressure-volume diagram for the lungs during eupnea. Relative volume is plotted against transpulmonary pressure difference, P_{TP}. The straight line is the static compliance curve for the lungs, ignoring hysteresis. We see that for any given volume change, P_{TP} must change significantly more during dynamic breathing than during the static situation, except at end-inspiration and end-expiration. At these points airflow stops for an instant. These augmented P_{TP} changes are required for overcoming airway and tissue resistances.

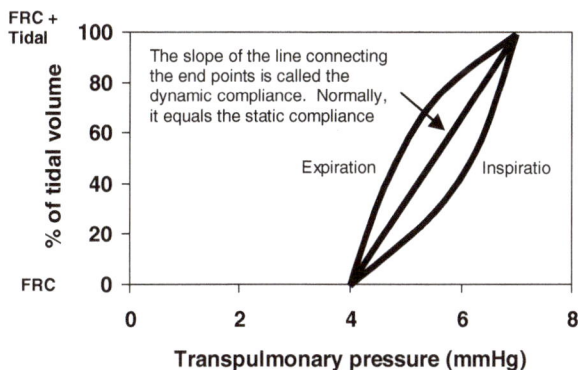

Figure 6. Dynamic pressure-volume loop over the range of a normal tidal volume.

The slope of the straight line connecting the end-expiratory pressure-volume point with the end-inspiratory pressure-volume point is often called "dynamic compliance" although this is somewhat of a misnomer. In the normal situation shown in Figure 6, "dynamic compliance" equals static compliance.

Topic 2: Time Constants and the Effect of Breathing Frequency on Dynamic Compliance

A sudden change in transpulmonary pressure causes a quick, but not instantaneous change in lung volume. The change in lung volume is an exponential function of time. The time required for 63% of the total change in volume is called the time constant. If pulmonary time constants were long enough to compare to the times available for inspiration and expiration, then lung inflation might be incomplete by the time expiration begins and deflation might be incomplete by the time the next inspiration begins. Normally, the time constants for

the pulmonary system are so short that even at high frequencies of breathing inflation and deflation are easily completed in the time available. This may not be true in obstructive pulmonary disorders.

Figure 7
An increase in static compliance can increase the time constants for inflation and deflation simply because more air is moved for any given change in intrapleural pressure, and this takes time. Increased airway resistance also increases the time constants since for any given change in transairway pressure, increased resistance slows the flow. This is exactly the situation in emphysema: high static compliance and high airway resistance. Consequently, emphysema can cause incomplete inflation during inspiration and incomplete deflation during expiration. The effect is to rotate the dynamic compliance loop clockwise as seen in Figure 7.

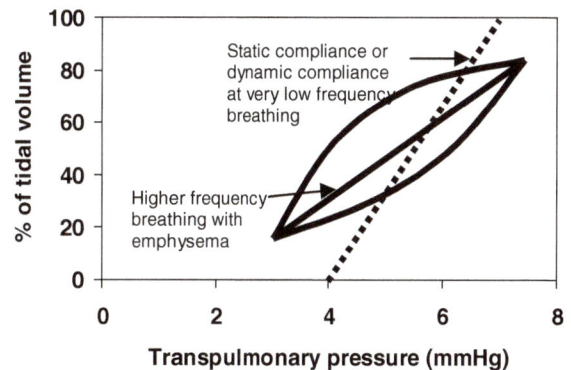

Figure 7. Clockwise rotation of dynamic compliance loop in emphysema at fairly high frequency breathing.

Figure 8
This effect of emphysema is usually not apparent at low breathing frequencies, but at higher frequencies when the times available are reduced, inflation and deflation may be aborted prematurely, elevating end-expiratory volume and depressing end-inspiratory volume. The effect of breathing frequency on dynamic compliance (as defined above) is shown in Figure 8. There is no appreciable effect of frequency on dynamic compliance in normal people. In patients with obstructive pulmonary diseases, however, dynamic compliance progressively decreases as breathing frequency increases. This effect can be enormous. Measurements of dynamic compliance can be a more sensitive clinical test for emphysema than simply measuring airway resistance (see below).

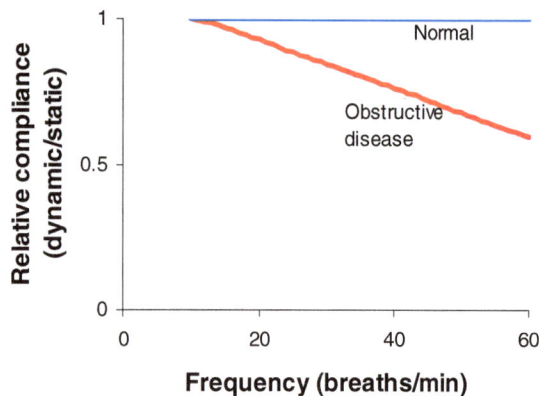

Figure 8. Effect of breathing frequency on the ratio of dynamic compliance to static compliance. Static compliance, of course, does not change with frequency, so the entire effect on the ratio in patients with obstructive lung disorders is due to decreased dynamic compliance.

Part 4: Airway Resistance

Topic 1: Definition and Measurement

Airway resistance (R_{AW}) is defined by the ratio of pressure difference to flow rate ($\dot{V}$):

$$R_{AW} = \frac{P_A - P_{AO}}{\dot{V}}$$

Measurement of R_{AW} requires measurement of $\dot{V}$ and P_A. $\dot{V}$ is easily measured with a flow meter (pneumotachometer) in the breathing tube. Measurement of P_A is more difficult and requires body plethysmography. The subject breaths box air rather than outside air. When the subject inhales, pressure in the box tends to increase due to increased thoracic volume, but tends to decrease due to removal of inhaled air. Which effect is the greater? Remember that alveolar pressure goes down during inspiration. This means that the number of air molecules inhaled is less than the number that are displaced in the box by the expanding thorax, and the box pressure increases. There is a calibration technique that can convert changes in box pressure to values for alveolar pressure, but at this point, you probably don't need to know the details.

Topic 2: Distribution of Airway Resistance

About 50% of total airway resistance is in the upper airways (nose to larynx). Most of the other 50% is in the trachea and large bronchi. Only about 10% of total R_{AW} is in airways having diameters less than about 2-3 mm. Now here is an important caveat. Obstruction of smaller airways can easily go unnoticed when total airway resistance is measured. In fact, complete obstruction of small airways leading to 50% of all alveoli will only increase R_{AW} by about 10%. So don't be misled by PFT data on R_{AW}.

Effect of Branching

Branching increases the number of parallel paths but decreases the diameter of each. Theoretically, branching can increase total resistance to flow, or decrease it depending on the number and diameters of the downstream paths. In the cardiovascular system, arterial branching increases total resistance until maximum resistance is attained at the level of arterioles. In the pulmonary system, the parallel branches are more numerous than in the arterial system and successive branching results in successively <u>less</u> total resistance to flow.

Topic 3: Factors that Normally Influence Airway Resistance

Flow Patterns in Airways

Laminar Flow

In laminar flow through tubes, concentric, molecularly thin layers of fluid pass over each other at velocities that progressively increase from rim to central axis. At any point, speed and direction are constant. Laminar flow is efficient; the pressure head required for a given flow rate is small compared to turbulent flow. Laminar flow is also quiet – there are no vibrations. Seems idyllic. Laminar flow is the rule in the cardiovascular system, but unfortunately, in the pulmonary system laminar flow is only present in very small airways. Elsewhere in the airway system, conditions are not right for laminar flow and either turbulent flow or transitional flow dominates.

Resistance is least in laminar flow. In addition, resistance is not influenced by flow rate. In other words, Ohm's Law is obeyed.

Turbulent Flow

The equation for the Reynolds number (Re) shows the variables that determine whether viscous flow will be laminar or turbulent:

$$\mathrm{Re} = \frac{\bar{v}\,\rho\,r}{\eta}$$

where $\bar{v}$ = mean velocity, ρ = density, r = tube radius, and η = viscosity.

The higher the Reynolds number the more likely is turbulent flow. Little eddies are always trying to disturb laminar flow and if Re gets too high, eddies can take over, breaking up the idyllic laminar pattern into chaotic swirls. We see from the Reynolds equation that increased flow velocity, increased air density, increased airway radius, and decreased air viscosity all increase the probability of turbulence. In many viscous flow situations, there is a critical Re, above which turbulence is likely. Perhaps you recall that for blood flow through straight tubes the critical Re is about 1000. It is not appropriate to state a critical Reynolds number for the intrathoracic airways due to all the branching and surface irregularity. Many textbooks use the value of 1000, but in reality, turbulence can develop in the airways at a Re as low as 1.0. Presumably, in the trachea the critical Re is closer to 1000.

Resistance is greatest in turbulent flow, and increasing the flow rate increases it even more. In laminar flow $\dot{V} \propto \Delta P$. In turbulent flow $\dot{V} \propto \sqrt{\Delta P}$. This relationship for turbulent flow is not very accurate, but it tells us that for a given flow rate, the driving pressure must be much greater for turbulent flow than for laminar flow.

Laminar flow exists in small bronchioles because velocity is very low (due to large total cross sectional area), and radius of each tube is small. Turbulent flow dominates in the upper airways. Transitional flow is in between.

Transitional (Disturbed) Flow

Transitional flow is not well defined. There are eddies at branches and these eddies may travel for some distance beyond the branches, but then resolve into laminar flow again. This situation dominates in most of the bronchi and bronchioles. Resistance is higher than it is with laminar flow, but lower than it is with truly turbulent flow.

Airway Caliber

We have just seen that the type of flow regime importantly influences airway resistance. Turbulent, transitional, and laminar flows blend into each other as the airways are descended. The other major determinant of airway resistance is the caliber (diameter) of the airways.

Do you remember the Poiseuille equation? In case you don't, it tells us that resistance through a single tube during laminar flow is given by:

$$R = \frac{8\,\eta\,l}{\pi\,r^4}$$

where η is viscosity, l is length, and r is radius

Viscosity changes are not important; neither are length changes. The really important thing here is radius. If radius decreases by a paltry 5%, R increases by 23%

The Poiseuille equation is valid for laminar flow of an incompressible Newtonian liquid through a straight, rigid, cylindrical tube. Obviously, these qualifications do not hold for the airways, but the r^4 rule is still roughly true, at least during laminar flow, and is useful for understanding the effects of changes in airway dimensions. The bottom line is that airway radius is very important.

Airway Smooth Muscle

Flow regimes cannot be adjusted directly by neurohumoral mechanisms, although their spatial ranges change with the intensity of breathing. But neurohumoral mechanisms are extremely important in adjusting airway calibers since they regulate airway smooth muscle contraction.

Effects of the Autonomic Nervous System and Circulating Epinephrine

- Parasympathetic activity, acting on muscarinic cholinergic receptors, promotes smooth muscle contraction, and therefore decreases airway caliber and increases airway resistance. [This is not an in-depth discussion of airway smooth muscle physiology, so mechanisms will not be covered.]

- Airway smooth muscle membranes are richly endowed with β_2 adrenergic receptors, which when activated result in airway smooth muscle relaxation (the same as with vascular smooth muscle). However, airway smooth muscle is not controlled much by direct sympathetic nerve activity; there are three reasons for this: 1) sympathetic innervation of airway smooth muscle is very sparse, 2) norepinephrine has virtually no effect on β_2 receptors, and 3) α_1 receptors on airway smooth muscle, which promote contraction, are not abundant. Circulating epinephrine (adrenalin) from the adrenal medulla is the main activator of β_2 adrenergic receptors on airway smooth muscle. Circulating epinephrine is an important dilator of airways in exercise, and in stressful situations. β_2 adrenergic agonists are extensively used for promoting bronchodilation.
- Nonadrenergic-noncholinergic (NANC) inhibitory nerve fibers run with the parasympathetic nerves. They release nitric oxide as the neurotransmitter. Nitric oxide causes relaxation of airway smooth muscle, and therefore decreased airway resistance by the same mechanism that is does in vascular smooth muscle.
- NANC stimulatory fibers are also present, but their role in regulating airway resistance is not clear.

Effects of Other Agents

Histamine constricts airway smooth muscle. So do some prostaglandins. Other prostaglandins relax airway smooth muscle. Chemical irritants, smoke, and dust can cause reflex constriction of airways. Decreased partial pressure of O_2 or increased partial pressure of CO_2 in inspired air or in particular regions of the airway system can cause generalized or local airway dilation. The pharmacology of airway smooth muscle is extraordinarily important, but more than this brief account is beyond the scope of a chapter on mechanics.

Lung Volume
Figure 9
As lung volume increases, the caliber of intrathoracic airways increases and airway resistance goes down. This is a very large effect

when going all the way from residual volume to total lung capacity, as shown in Figure 9. Even during eupnea, the effect is appreciable. It is caused, of course, by expansion of all hollow places in the lungs during inspiration and compression during expiration. Not only do the alveoli follow this routine, but also (to a lesser degree) the airways. When intrapleural pressure decreases, everything expands; when it increases, everything compresses. Notice that the effect on R_{AW} is much steeper at lung volumes below FRC than above FRC.

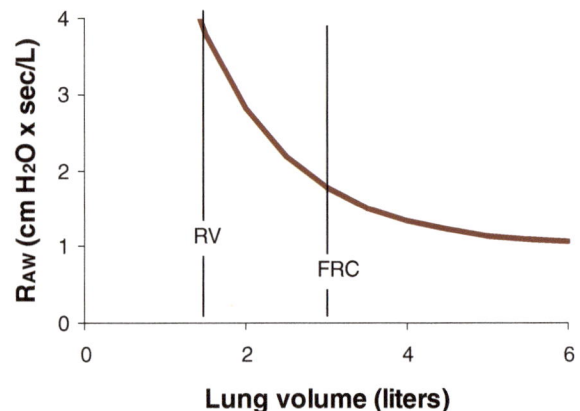

Figure 9. Effect of lung volume on airway resistance, R_{AW}. From G. Sant'Ambrogio and F.B. Sant'Ambrogio, Mechanics of Breathing: Statics, in *The Medical Physiology and Biophysics Syllabus*, UTMB, 1998.

Two forces determine the caliber of intrathoracic airways during changes in lung volume: 1) the transmural pressure change *per se*, and 2) the pull on the airways by fibrous connections with their surroundings. The latter force is called radial traction. As intrapleural pressure decreases during inspiration, an increase in transmural pressure across the intrathoracic airways together with an increase in radial traction opens the intrathoracic airways and R_{AW} decreases. The opposite happens during expiration.

Dynamic Compression of Airways during Forced Expiration
During normal eupneic breathing, translung pressure (P_L) is always positive; *i.e.* alveolar pressure remains greater than intrapleural pressure throughout the breathing cycle (see Figure 12 of Chapter 2). This is mainly because intrapleural pressure remains negative throughout the breathing cycle. For the same reason, transmural pressure across the intrathoracic airways is always positive

during normal quiet breathing and the airways are kept distended. With a forced expiration, however, something curious happens. A forced expiration can raise intrapleural pressure to as much as +120 cm of water (90 mmHg). Alveolar pressure rises accordingly and air is forcefully exhaled. The distending pressure across the alveolar walls (P_L) remains positive and the alveoli remain open. But what happens to pressure in the airways as air rapidly flows out? Airway pressure progressively drops because of viscous resistance until finally it reaches zero at the airway opening. Somewhere along the way, airway pressure drops enough to equal intrapleural pressure. This location is called the equal pressure point (EPP). Beyond the EPP (toward the mouth) airway pressure drops below intrapleural pressure creating a compression force on the airways. At low lung volumes, this pressure reversal can take place in airways that are small enough not to be held open strongly by cartilage; these airways can completely collapse, temporarily preventing airflow through them. When airflow stops, pressure in the airways leading to the EPP rises until it exceeds intrapleural pressure – the airways then open again allowing flow to occur, but as soon as flow is reestablished, the pressure drops again and the airways are compressed again. So they flutter. Now a curious thing is that during the fluttering process, the pressure difference that determines the rate of airflow is no longer P_A - P_{AO}, but now is P_A - P_{PL}. At high lung volumes, the airways are open wider, and the EPP is located farther up into the region of cartilaginous rings and compression is resisted.

Figure 10

There is another curious thing. Figure 10 plots the rate of airflow as a function of the change in lung volume during forced expirations. The procedure starts at total lung capacity (TLC) and forced expiration continues all the way down to residual volume (RV). In other words, the entire vital capacity is exhaled. Expiratory flow rate reaches a maximal value rather quickly and then declines gradually, finally reaching zero at RV. The different curves are for different intensities of expiratory effort. The curious thing is that as RV is approached the curve becomes independent of effort – it is essentially the same at maximal effort as it is at less than maximal effort. The first part of the curve (at high lung volumes) is effort-dependent, but the part of the curve at low lung volumes is effort-independent. The reason effort doesn't matter during expiration at low lung

volumes is that P_A - P_{PL} isn't influenced by effort at low lung volumes; P_A and P_{PL} are both elevated the same amount by increased expiratory effort. Since flow rate is determined by P_A - P_{PL} during dynamic airway collapse, it is effort-independent.

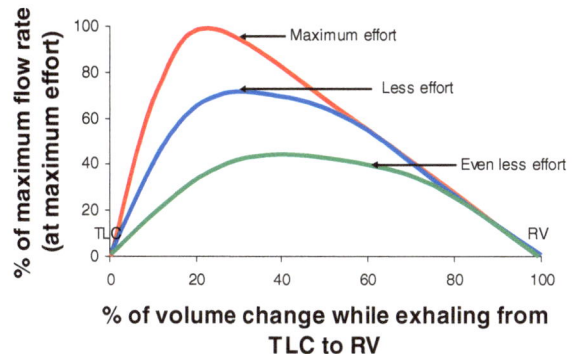

Figure 10. Flow-volume curves at varying intensities of expiratory effort.

Topic 4: Disease and Airway Resistance

Two major categories of generalized pulmonary disease are recognized: obstructive and restrictive. They both involve changes in airway resistance.

Obstructive pulmonary diseases include asthma, bronchiectasis, emphysema, and chronic bronchitis. The latter two are called chronic obstructive pulmonary disease, COPD. Obstructive diseases are characterized by increased RV, FRC, TLC, and to a lesser degree VC. There is increased lower airway resistance, and major difficulty in expiring. In emphysema, there is extensive destruction of interstitial elastic fibers with greatly reduced radial traction on the small airways. Consequently, dynamic airway collapse during expiration can be a major problem. 'Pursing' the lips and partially closing the glottis during expiration can help by raising airway pressure.

Restrictive pulmonary diseases include a large number of conditions.
- Some reduce lung compliance (*e.g.* pulmonary fibrosis, sarcoidosis, congestive heart failure, pneumonia, and various pneumoconioses and infiltrative conditions)
- Some reduce thoracic compliance (*e.g.* obesity, pleural diseases, fibrothorax, kyphoscoliosis, and aging)

- Some reduce the ability of the muscles of inspiration to expand the thorax (neuromuscular disorders).

Restrictive diseases are characterized by reduced RV, FRC, TLC, and VC, increased lower airway resistance, and major difficulty in <u>inspiring</u>. In restrictive pulmonary diseases, airway resistance is increased, but only to the extent that lung volume is decreased (see Figure 9).

Figure 11
Flow-volume curves have rather characteristic patterns in obstructive and restrictive diseases as shown in Figure 11.

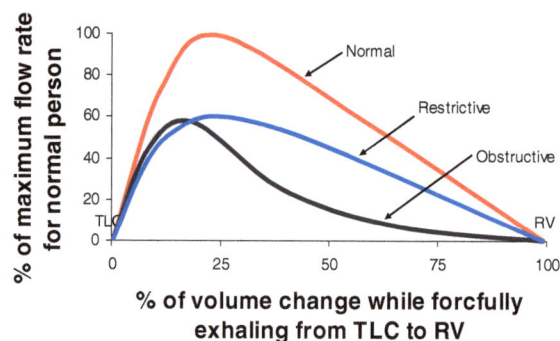

Figure 11. Flow-volume curves typical of obstructive and restrictive pulmonary diseases compared to normal, all at maximum effort.

Part 5: Regional Variations in Alveolar Ventilation

In a supine posture, at FRC, the alveoli are inflated to about the same degree at the apex of the lungs as they are at the base. Consequently, they have about the same compliance and upon inspiration they fill to about the same degree. However, in an upright posture, again at FRC, the alveoli near the apex are inflated more than they are in the supine position and those near the base are inflated less. In fact, the alveoli near the apex are so large that their compliance is reduced (*i.e.* further inflation is difficult). Thus, there is a progressive increase in alveolar compliance from apex to base. Consequently, upon inspiration there is a progressive increase in alveolar ventilation from apex to base.

There is also a gradient in intrapleural pressure. In an upright posture, either standing or sitting, P_{PL} is most negative near the apex of the lungs and least negative near the base.

Similar gradients at FRC can be seen in people who are lying on their side, except that now the gradients run from the top side to the bottom side of the lungs rather than from apex to base. This observation demonstrates that the alveolar inflation and P_{PL} gradients are at least partly caused by gravity.

Just how gravity causes these two gradients is not entirely clear. Some authors give vague explanations related to the weight of the lung parenchyma, the weight of the fluid in the intrapleural space, or the weight of pulmonary blood. It is also not clear whether the decrease in P_{PL} near the apex causes the increase in alveolar volume or *vice versa*.

Since in an upright posture the alveoli near the top of the lungs are already considerably inflated at FRC and those near the base are considerably deflated, those near the top contribute most of the expiratory reserve volume (ERV) and those nearer the base account for most of the inspiratory reserve volume (IRV).

Part 6: The Work of Breathing

During inspiration, energy must be expended to overcome two things:
1. <u>Elastic recoil</u> of the lungs (also the chest wall at high lung volumes)
2. <u>Frictional resistance</u> in the airways and tissues

Figure 12
It is customary to picture the work of inspiration using a pressure-volume diagram. The straight line in Figure 12 represents the static pressure-volume relationship (no air moving) over a normal tidal range. The curves represent the dynamic pressure-volume relationship. Perhaps you remember that pressure-volume work is given by the area under a

pressure-volume curve, measuring toward the volume axis. Thus, the crosshatched area equals the work required for overcoming elastic recoil during inspiration. The shaded area between the static line and the dynamic inspiratory curve equals the work required for overcoming frictional resistance during inspiration. Clearly, during eupnea, frictional work is much less than elastic recoil work. During heavy breathing, frictional work increases greatly due to increased airflow, and can be even greater than elastic recoil work.

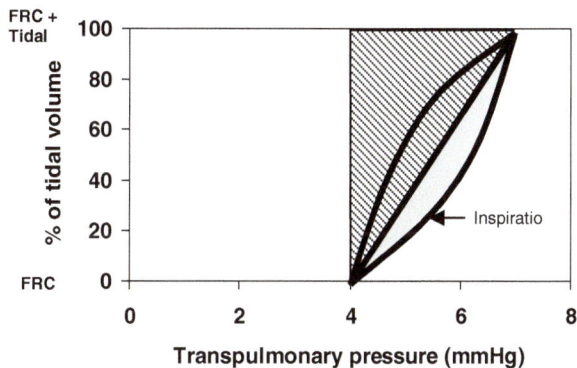

Figure 12. The work of inspiration. The crosshatched area is the work required to overcome elastic recoil of the lungs, including surface tension. The shaded area is the additional work required to overcome frictional resistance, especially flow resistance.

Remember that in normal breathing at rest, no work is required for expiration. In moderate to heavy exercise, however, and in obstructive pulmonary diseases, the work of expiration can become significant. Some authors have suggested ways of calculating the work of expiration from dynamic expiratory pressure-volume curves, but they have never made much sense to me.

During normal breathing at rest, the muscles of respiration use about 3-5% of total-body oxygen consumption. During exercise, this percentage can rise markedly.

Restrictive pulmonary diseases increase elastic recoil work and can also increase tissue resistance. Obstructive pulmonary diseases increase the work required for overcoming airway resistance and, in the case of emphysema, can actually reduce recoil work.

Figure 13

In emphysema, the work of breathing (measured here as oxygen consumption by the respiratory muscles) is increased above normal even at resting levels of ventilation (about 6-10 liters/min). But far more dramatic is the huge increase in oxygen consumption required for increasing the rate of ventilation.

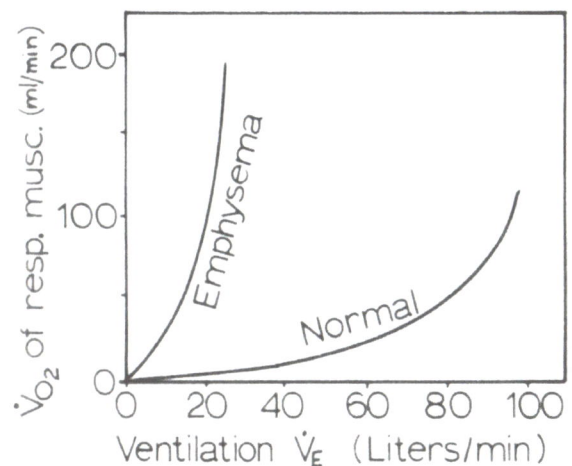

Figure 13. The rate of oxygen consumption by the respiratory muscles as a function of the rate of ventilation. A patient with emphysema is compared to a normal person. From T.C. Ruch and H.D. Patton, Physiology and Biophysics, 19th Ed., Saunders, 1965.

Chapter 4

Alveolar Ventilation

Part 1: Principles of Alveolar Ventilation
Part 2: Composition of Air in the Lower Airways and Alveoli
Part 3: Causes of Abnormally Low Alveolar PO$_2$
Part 4: Typical Normal Values
Part 5: What Can Go Wrong?

Part 1: Principles of Alveolar Ventilation

Topic 1: Introduction

The pulmonary air spaces can be divided into conducting airways and alveoli. The branching tree of conducting airways extends from mouth and nose to the terminal bronchioles, then on to the respiratory bronchioles from which bud a limited number of alveoli. The respiratory bronchioles together with their alveoli are a transitional region having a limited capacity for gas exchange with blood. The respiratory bronchioles lead to the alveolar ducts and sacs, which are loaded with alveoli. Almost all gas exchange between pulmonary air and blood occurs across the walls of alveoli. For simplicity we generally ignore the transition region and consider the pulmonary spaces to consist of conducting airways with no capacity for gas exchange and alveoli in which all gas exchange is accomplished.

[Note: The important equations in this chapter are numbered. The others are transitional, mostly involved with derivations. Most readers will probably not be very interested in learning the derivations, but they could help understanding.]

Topic 2: Dead Space and Alveolar Space

Anatomic Dead Space
Since no gas exchange occurs in the conducting airways their contained volume is called the anatomic dead space. The anatomic dead space in a normal person is roughly 1 ml per pound of body weight. So a normal 150 lb person would have about 150 ml of dead space. When this person inhales a tidal volume of 500 ml, only 350 ml reach the alveoli, the other 150 ml do not get past the dead space. Total tidal volume, V_T, is split between dead space volume (V_D) and alveolar volume (V_A).

$$V_T = V_D + V_A \qquad (1)$$

V_T can be directly measured by spirometry, and V_A can then be calculated as V_T - V_D.

[Note: In this discussion, V_A is not the total alveolar gas volume; it is that portion of tidal volume that enters or leaves the alveoli.]

Consider a person who is panting with a tidal volume of only 150 ml. Inspiring 150 ml is only enough to fill the dead space with none left over for the alveoli, so there is no gas exchange between incoming air and blood and the subject could asphyxiate. On the other hand, consider a person trying to breathe through a long garden hose. Inspiration and expiration of a normal tidal volume would only move air through the dead space (his own dead space plus that of the garden hose) and, again, he would asphyxiate. [There was once a Dick Tracy cartoon strip in which the arch enemy, Flat Top, avoided capture by submerging himself in a river and breathing in and out through a long garden hose – not possible.]

Measurement of Anatomic Dead Space
The rough rule of 1 ml/lb of body weight may not be good enough, so there is a more accurate clinical measurement that can be performed. It is called the Fowler method and is quite simple. The patient takes a single inspiration of 100% oxygen and then breathes out. The outgoing air passes through a nitrogen analyzer. As the dead space air goes out, the nitrogen reading is zero since it is 100% oxygen. Subsequently, as alveolar air goes out, the nitrogen concentration increases and quickly reaches the nitrogen concentration present in alveolar air. The volume exhaled to the point at which nitrogen concentration is roughly half its

final value is taken to be the volume of the anatomic dead space.

Physiologic Dead Space

In certain abnormal situations there are some ventilated alveoli that accomplish no gas exchange with blood. This can happen, for example, when blood flow is blocked to some alveoli by a pulmonary embolus. Ventilated alveoli that have no blood flow and, therefore, no gas exchange contribute to dead space. This contribution is called alveolar dead space. Anatomic dead space plus alveolar dead space is called physiologic dead space. Normally, there is almost no alveolar dead space and physiologic dead space is practically the same as anatomic dead space.

Measurement of Physiologic Dead Space and Functional Alveolar Space

When there is an appreciable alveolar dead space the tidal volume (V_T) is given by

$$V_T = V_{Dp} + V_{Af} \qquad (2)$$

- V_{Dp} = physiologic dead space
- V_{Af} = functional alveolar space

The functional alveolar space (*i.e.* the gas-exchanging alveolar space) can be measured by the following CO_2 dilution method. There is essentially no CO_2 in inspired air and, therefore, at the end of inspiration there is no CO_2 in dead space air. So any CO_2 that appears in expired air must have come from functional alveoli. If we measure the amount of CO_2 in a tidal expiration and divide by the concentration of CO_2 in functional alveoli we get the volume of air exhaled from functional alveoli (amount/concentration = volume).

$$V_{Af} = \frac{V_E CO_2}{F_{Af} CO_2} \qquad (3)$$

- V_{Af} = volume of functional alveolar space exhaled in a single breath
- $V_E CO_2$ = volume of CO_2 exhaled in a single breath
- $F_{Af} CO_2$ the fractional concentration of CO_2 in the functional alveolar space

The only problem is determining alveolar CO_2 concentration. This can be done by measuring CO_2 concentration in expired air at the end of a normal

tidal volume since at this point only alveolar air is being exhaled. Alternatively, alveolar CO_2 concentration can be obtained from arterial blood gas analysis since arterial P_{CO_2} is nearly always the same as alveolar P_{CO_2}. The first method suffers from the fact that when alveolar dead space is large, CO_2 from functional alveoli is appreciably diluted by air from non-functional alveoli. The second method is usually better, but cannot be used when there is a large venous-to-arterial shunt since then $P_A CO_2$ is less than $PaCO_2$.

[Note: The indicator-dilution principle for determining volumes is extremely important in many clinical measurements, including the Fick, dye dilution, and thermal dilution methods for cardiac output, the dye dilution method for plasma volume, and many others including in this case, V_{Af}.]

Of course, the physiologic dead space, V_{Dp}, can be obtained simply by subtracting V_{Af} from V_T

$$V_{Dp} = V_T - \frac{V_E CO_2}{F_{Af} CO_2}$$

This is all we really need to calculate physiologic dead space, but wait, there's more. We know that

$$V_E CO_2 = F_E CO_2 \times V_T$$

Therefore

$$V_{Dp} = V_T - \frac{F_E CO_2 \times V_T}{F_{Af} CO_2}$$

Rearranging we get

$$V_{Dp} = V_T \frac{F_{Af} CO_2 - F_E CO_2}{F_{Af} CO_2}$$

- $F_{Af} CO_2$ = fractional CO_2 concentration in functional alveoli
- $F_E CO_2$ = fractional CO_2 concentration in mixed expired air

Now we multiply fractional concentrations by barometric pressure to get

$$V_{Dp} = V_T \frac{P_{Af} CO_2 - P_E CO_2}{P_{Af} CO_2} \qquad (4)$$

- $P_{Af}CO_2 = PCO_2$ in functional alveolar air
- $P_ECO_2 = PCO_2$ in mixed expired air (expired dead space air mixed with expired alveolar air)

Equation 4 is called the <u>Bohr equation</u>. It is often used for determining physiologic dead space. $P_{Af}CO_2$ can be estimated either from end-expiratory gas or from $PaCO_2$ as discussed above.

Topic 3: Ventilation

If the single breath volumes discussed above are multiplied by the breathing frequency in breaths/min we get <u>minute ventilation</u>. For example, V_T x frequency = total minute ventilation (usually in liters/min). The symbol for minute ventilation, whether total, dead space, or alveolar is $\dot{V}$ (pronounced V dot).

Thus we have:

$\dot{V}_I$ for volume inspired per minute

$\dot{V}_E$ for volume exhaled per minute

$\dot{V}_D$ for dead space ventilation per minute

$\dot{V}_A$ for alveolar ventilation per minute

$\dot{V}_E$ is usually a little less than $\dot{V}_I$ owing to the fact that the rate of CO_2 production by metabolism is usually less than the rate of O_2 consumption. By convention we use $\dot{V}_E$ rather than $\dot{V}_I$ for total minute ventilation.

The ventilation equivalent of Equation 1 is:

$$\dot{V}_E = \dot{V}_D + \dot{V}_A \qquad (5)$$

A normal resting person might have a V_E of 500 ml, a V_D of 150 ml, and a breathing frequency of 12/min. In this case

$\dot{V}_E = 6.0$ L/min

$\dot{V}_D = 1.8$ L/min

$\dot{V}_A = 4.2$ L/min

Effect of Breathing Frequency on Alveolar Ventilation

Equation 5 can be modified by substituting

$V_D \times frequency$ for $\dot{V}_D$. After solving for $\dot{V}_A$ we have

$$\dot{V}_A = \dot{V}_E - V_D \times frequency$$

Figure 1

Figure 1 is a plot of $\dot{V}_A$ as a function of frequency assuming that $\dot{V}_E$ and V_D remain constant. With increasing frequency, more and more of the tidal volume is used for ventilating dead space and less for ventilating alveoli until finally there is no alveolar ventilation at all.

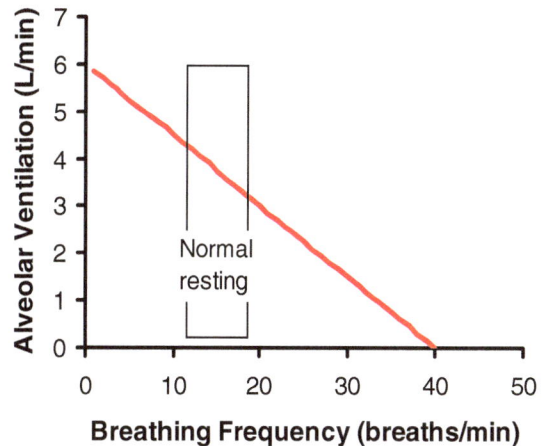

Figure 1. Effect of breathing frequency on alveolar ventilation. Total minute ventilation assumed constant at 6.0 L/min. Dead space assumed constant at 150 ml.

In mechanical ventilation, relatively large tidal volumes are used at relatively low frequencies maintaining a normal $\dot{V}_E$. Thus, the ratio of $\dot{V}_A$ to $\dot{V}_E$ is increased. On the other hand, at very high frequencies but low tidal volumes, $\dot{V}_A$ can be normal but there is greatly increased $\dot{V}_D$. This kind of breathing, panting, is used by dogs for getting rid of body heat.

Regional Variations in Alveolar Ventilation

In an upright posture, the alveoli near the top (apex) of the lungs are ventilated less than the alveoli near the bottom (base) of the lungs. This phenomenon results from the fact that the apical alveoli are already fairly well inflated before inspiration begins while the basal alveoli are somewhat deflated. This regional variation in ventilation was discussed in Part 5 of Chapter 3 and will be important later when we study the ratio of alveolar ventilation to alveolar blood flow, the $\dot{V}/\dot{Q}$ ratio.

Part 2: Composition of Air in the Lower Airways and Alveoli

Topic 1: Lower Airways

During Inspiration

As inspired air passes through the upper airways (defined as everything down to the larynx) it is quickly warmed to body temperature and saturated with water vapor. At body temperature the water vapor pressure is 47 mmHg. This translates to an addition of about 6.2 ml of water vapor for every 100 ml of dry air inspired. Thus, the O_2 and N_2 in inspired dry air are diluted about 6% by water vapor.

After humidification,

$$P_I O_2 + P_I N_2 = P_B - P_I water$$

P_B = barometric (atmospheric) pressure)

We know the ratio of O_2 volume to N_2 volume in dry air and from this information we can determine that after humidification

$$P_I O_2 = F_I O_2 \times (P_B - P_{water}) \qquad (6)$$

$F_I O_2$ in this equation is the fractional oxygen concentration in <u>dry</u> air.

So at sea level $P_I O_2$ is given by

$$P_I O_2 = 0.21 \times (760 - 47) = 150 \; mmHg$$

Therefore, humidified inspired air in the dead space consists of O_2 at 150 mmHg, H_2O at 47 mmHg, and N_2 at 563 mmHg. The fractional concentrations come out to be $O_2 = 0.20$, $H_2O = 0.06$, and $N_2 = 0.74$.

At End-Expiration

At the end of expiration of a normal tidal volume the composition of air in the dead space is the same as that in alveolar air.

Topic 2: Alveoli

Carbon Dioxide

A normal 150 lb person at rest generates roughly 240 ml of CO_2 per minute. In the steady state, this same volume of CO_2 must be exhaled per minute. All of the exhaled CO_2 comes from the alveoli. If this person's $\dot{V}_E CO_2$ is 240 ml/min, and $\dot{V}_A$ is 4500 ml/min, the fractional concentration of CO_2 in alveolar air must have been 240 ml/4500 ml = 0.053 since concentration equals amount/volume. So alveolar air is ordinarily about 5.3% CO_2. Notice that this is simply another application of the CO_2 dilution equation, in this case solved for $F_A CO_2$.

$$F_A CO_2 = \frac{\dot{V}_E CO_2}{\dot{V}_A}$$

At an atmospheric pressure of 760 mmHg, 5.3% CO_2 is equivalent to about 40 mmHg (760 x 0.053). Notice from the above equation that if alveolar ventilation increases with no change in CO_2 production, $F_A CO_2$ and, therefore $P_A CO_2$ decrease. An increase in $P_A CO_2$ above normal signifies hypoventilation. A decrease in $P_A CO_2$ signifies hyperventilation.

Oxygen

Our normal 150 lb person at rest consumes about 300 ml of O_2 per minute. The volume of O_2 inhaled/min must equal the volume of O_2 consumed/min plus that which ventilates the dead space and the alveolar space. Therefore,

$$\dot{V}_I \times F_I O_2 = \dot{V} O_2 + \dot{V}_D \times F_D O_2 + \dot{V}_A \times F_A O_2$$

- The term on the left is the volume of O_2 inhaled/min (total volume inspired/min x fractional concentration of O_2 in <u>humidified</u> inspired air).
- The first term on the right is the volume of O_2 consumed by metabolism per minute.
- The second term on the right is the volume of O_2 ventilating the dead space/min.
- The third term on the right is the volume of O_2 ventilating the alveoli/min.

Solving for $F_A O_2$ and substituting $\dot{V}_A = \dot{V}_I - \dot{V}_D$ we get:

$$F_A O_2 = F_I O_2 - \frac{\dot{V} O_2}{\dot{V}_A} \qquad (7)$$

If O_2 consumption is 300 ml/min, and alveolar ventilation is 4500 ml/min, and the fractional concentration of O_2 in humidified inspired air is 0.20, then the fractional concentration of O_2 in alveoli is 0.13. Thus, $P_A O_2$ is nearly 100 mmHg, or about 2.5 times that of CO_2. The above equation shows that as alveolar ventilation increases, the concentration of O_2 in alveolar air increases, but can only increase to the concentration in inspired air.

Figure 2
The effects of changing alveolar ventilation on $P_A CO_2$ and $P_A O_2$ are shown in Figure 2.

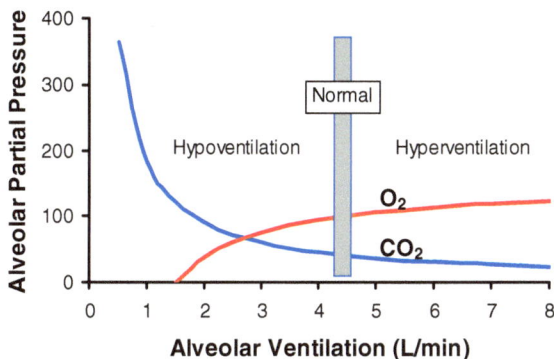

Figure 2. Effects of changing alveolar ventilation on $P_A O_2$ and $P_A CO_2$. It is assumed that the rates of O_2 consumption and CO_2 production remain constant.

The Alveolar Air Equation
But can $P_A O_2$ be calculated without knowing the rate of oxygen consumption or the rate of alveolar ventilation? The answer is yes, but you do need to know $P_A CO_2$. The calculation is made by using an important equation called the alveolar air equation (also called the alveolar gas equation). The alveolar air equation is:

$$P_A O_2 = P_I O_2 - \frac{P_A CO_2}{R} + \left\{ P_A CO_2 \times F_I O_2 \times \left(\frac{1}{R} - 1 \right) \right\}$$

The derivation of the alveolar air equation is complex and will not be given here. The term in brackets {} is only about 2 mmHg and is often ignored. Therefore, for simplicity, the equation is usually written as:

$$P_A O_2 = P_I O_2 - \frac{P_A CO_2}{R} \qquad (8)$$

$P_I O_2$ is for humidified inspired air and is given by Equation 6, $P_I O_2 = F_I O_2 \times \left(P_B - P_{water} \right)$.

Therefore, another form of the alveolar air equation is:

$$P_A O_2 = F_I O_2 \times \left(P_B - P_{water} \right) - \frac{P_A CO_2}{R} \qquad (9)$$

- $F_I O_2$ is the fractional O_2 concentration in dry ambient air (= 0.21)
- P_B is total barometric (ambient) pressure and is 760 mmHg at sea level. It decreases with increasing altitude.
- P_{water} is the vapor pressure of water in humidified air at body temperature. This value is 47 mmHg and is not influenced by barometric pressure.
- R is the respiratory exchange ratio (often called the respiratory quotient, RQ). This is the ratio of CO_2 production to O_2 consumption and is usually about 0.80 for a person on an ordinary mixed diet. If only carbohydrates are consumed $R = 1.0$. If only fat is consumed $R = 0.7$.

$P_A CO_2$ can be measured by analyzing end-expiratory gas or, since $P_A CO_2 \approx PaCO_2$, replaced with a measured value of $PaCO_2$.

The alveolar air equation has been very important in aviation for calculating the O_2 concentration necessary to deliver *via* a breathing mask in order to get a satisfactory P_AO_2 at any particular altitude. This equation can also be used to calculate the cabin pressure necessary for a satisfactory P_AO_2.

In medical pulmonology, the alveolar air equation is used, together with arterial blood gas analysis, to determine the difference between P_AO_2 and PaO_2. This difference is called the A-a O_2 gradient. The A-a O_2 gradient is normally no greater than about 12 mmHg in young people. It can be abnormally large when there is a ventilation/perfusion mismatch (see Chapter 9) or when O_2 diffusion across the alveolar-capillary barrier is seriously impaired. With aging, the A-a O_2 gradient tends to increase. A rule of thumb is that the A-a O_2 gradient should not be larger than about age/4 + 4 mmHg. So a healthy 80 year-old person is expected to have an A-a O_2 gradient not larger than 24 mmHg.

Topic 3: Changes in P_ACO_2 and P_AO_2 during the Breathing Cycle

Of course, during inspiration P_ACO_2 decreases and P_AO_2 increases. The opposite happens during expiration. However, these fluctuations are not nearly as large as you might expect. This is largely due to the functional residual capacity, FRC, which in our normal 150 lb person is expected to be about 3.0 liters. This is a large volume compared to a normal alveolar intake of 350 ml in a single breath. Therefore, new alveolar air increases total alveolar air by less than 10 %. In addition, during the course of a single inhalation, some of the O_2 that enters alveoli diffuses on into capillary blood and doesn't build up in the alveoli. The result is that with a resting tidal volume of 500 ml, P_AO_2 varies around the mean of about 100 mmHg by only about 1 mmHg. A similar argument can be applied to P_ACO_2, which again varies during the breathing cycle by only about ± 1 mmHg. At higher tidal volumes, of course, these variations are greater.

Part 3: Causes of Abnormally Low P_AO_2

Low Barometric Pressure
The usual cause of abnormally low barometric pressure is ascent to high altitudes, either in an aircraft or by climbing a mountain. The alveolar air equation as given in Equation 9 predicts that as P_B decreases, P_AO_2 decreases as long as P_ACO_2 remains constant, *i.e.* no hyperventilation. For example, at an altitude of 15,000 ft, P_B is 429 mmHg. Plugging this value into Equation 8 reveals that P_AO_2 would only be 30 mmHg. Thus, the decline in P_AO_2 with increasing altitude is out of proportion to the decrease in atmospheric pressure. This much decline in P_AO_2 would lead to severe arterial hypoxemia, *i.e.* low PaO_2, which in turn would lead to activation of arterial chemoreceptors and hyperventilation (see Chapter 11). Thus, P_ACO_2 would decrease and P_AO_2 would return toward normal. For example, if P_ACO_2 dropped to 30 mmHg, P_AO_2 would rise to 38 mmHg.

Low Alveolar Ventilation
Another cause of low P_AO_2 is alveolar hypoventilation, which can result from a variety of neuromuscular disorders such as polio, amyotrophic lateral sclerosis, myasthenia gravis, *etc.* It can also result from increases in airway resistance due to chronic bronchitis, emphysema, asthma, *etc.*

Exercise
What about exercise? Oxygen consumption increases during exercise and you might think this would lower P_AO_2. But the rate of alveolar ventilation also increases during exercise to a degree that matches the increase in O_2 consumption.

The ratio $\dot{V}O_2 consumed / \dot{V}_A$ remains nearly constant and, therefore, F_AO_2 and P_AO_2 remain nearly constant over a wide range of exercise intensities. At very high exercise intensities P_AO_2 may actually rise moderately because of hyperventilation (lower alveolar CO_2 allows for higher alveolar O_2).

Part 4: Some Typical Normal Values

Fractional Concentrations and Partial Pressures			
Symbols	Description	Fractional Concentration	Corresponding Partial Pressure (mmHg)
F_IO_2 or P_IO_2	O_2 in dry inspired air	0.209	159
F_IO_2 or P_IO_2 (humidified)	O_2 in humidified inspired air (lower airways)	0.196	149
F_AO_2 or P_AO_2	O_2 in alveolar air	0.129	98
F_ICO_2 or P_ICO_2	CO_2 in inspired air	0.0003	0
F_ACO_2 or P_ACO_2	CO_2 in alveolar air	0.053	40
F_ECO_2 or P_ECO_2	CO_2 in mixed expired air	0.037	28
$F_A$water or $P_A$water	Water vapor in humidified air	0.062	47

Volumes and Rates			
Symbols	Description	Single Breath Volume (ml)	Minute volume at 12 breaths/min (ml/min)
V_T or $\dot{V}_E$	Tidal volume	500	6,000
V_D or $\dot{V}_D$	Dead space	150	1,800
V_A or $\dot{V}_A$	Alveolar volume	350	4,200

Others			
P_B	Barometric pressure	760 mmHg at sea level	
R	Respiratory exchange ratio (respiratory quotient)	0.7 to 1.0 Usually about 0.80 – 0.82	

Part 5: What Can Go Wrong?

The Causes of Hypoventilation

- Restrictive pulmonary diseases
  - Neuromuscular disorders
    - Amyotrophic lateral sclerosis
    - Polio
    - Muscular dystrophy
  - Interstitial pulmonary fibrosis
  - Scleroderma
  - Sarcoidosis
- Obstructive pulmonary diseases
  - Emphysema
  - Chronic bronchitis
  - Asthma
- Pneumothorax
- Drugs that cause respiratory depression (*e.g.* narcotics)

Chapter 5

Pulmonary Blood Flow and Fluid Balance

Part 1: The Pulmonary Circulation

Topic 1: Preliminaries

The pulmonary circulation is a low pressure, low resistance, and high compliance system.

Pulmonary artery pressure is quite low compared to aortic pressure, while pulmonary blood flow, of necessity, must equal systemic flow. This is possible because pulmonary vascular resistance is much lower than systemic vascular resistance. These comparisons are shown in Table 1.

Table 1	Pulmonary as % of Systemic
Mean arterial pressure	16%
Driving pressure (arterial – venous)	7%
Total resistance	7%
Flow rate	100%

Since afterload to the right ventricle (indicated by mean pulmonary artery pressure) is low, the right ventricle need not be very strong. Thus, its wall is relatively thin, and since it doesn't develop much tension it doesn't use much oxygen compared to the left ventricle.

Topic 2: Vascular Compliance

Pulmonary blood vessels are very distensible and can accommodate large increases in blood volume without much increase in pressure. This happens whenever we change from an erect posture to a reclining posture; some of the blood that runs out of the legs ends up in the lungs. Also, the pulmonary veins hold enough blood at a low pressure that they, together with the left atrium, provide a very important reservoir for rapid filling of the left ventricle during the early diastolic filling period (*i.e.* during diastolic suction).

Topic 3: Pulmonary Vascular Resistance (PVR)

Resistance to flow is defined as the driving pressure difference divided by the flow rate. For the pulmonary circulation

$$PVR = \frac{mPAP - mPVP}{CO}$$

$$PVR = pulmonary\ vascular\ resis\tan ce$$
$$mPAP = mean\ pulmonary\ artery\ pressure$$
$$mPVP = mean\ pulmonary\ vein\ pressure$$
$$CO = cardiac\ output$$

[If pressure is expressed in mmHg and flow in L/min, normal PVR is roughly 1.2 R units. This compares to 16 R units for the systemic circulation. The cgs system is often used; in this case normal PVR is about 100 dynes-sec/cm^5.]

Distribution of PVR

Total resistance in the pulmonary circulation is fairly evenly distributed among small arteries, capillaries, and small veins. In the systemic circulatory system, the arterioles account for roughly 65% of the total resistance to flow. This is because they are so narrow and muscular. Arterioles in the pulmonary system have larger diameters and are far less muscular. In fact, some authors prefer not to regard them as arterioles at all but rather as just small arteries. Nevertheless, as we shall see, these arterioles can constrict and have an important role in distributing blood flow preferentially to well ventilated alveoli that can use good blood flow and away from poorly ventilated alveoli that cannot use it. More about this a little later.

Effect of Intravascular Pressure on PVR and the Pressure-Flow Relationship

Most vascular beds in the body respond to increased driving pressure by an increase in resistance to flow. This property of <u>reactive</u> vascular beds is known as <u>pressure-flow autoregulation</u>. It results in a relatively constant flow rate over the usual range of driving pressures (the autoregulatory range). For example, blood flow to the brain is not seriously compromised until mean arterial pressure drops below about 60 mmHg. Approximately the same is true of the coronary, renal, intestinal, muscle, *etc.* circulations.

In contrast, the pulmonary vascular bed is not reactive, it is passive. It shows no pressure-flow autoregulation. Instead, when pressure in the pulmonary system increases the vessels simply expand and the resistance to flow decreases. In addition, increased pulmonary artery pressure results in recruitment of more capillaries (recruitment will be discussed later in this chapter). Consequently, resistance to flow decreases even more. The pressure-flow relationship for the pulmonary circulation is shown in Figure 1.

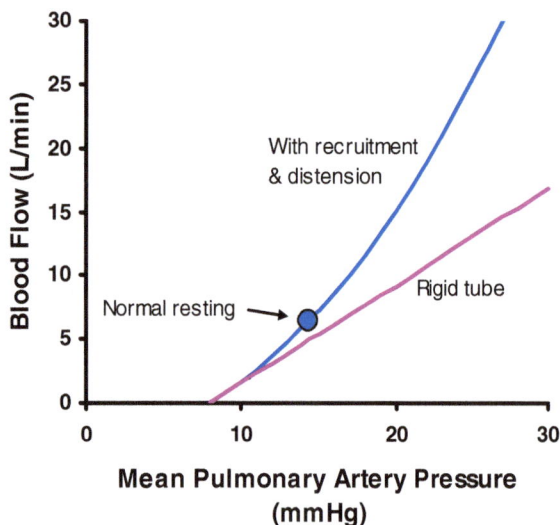

Figure 1. Pulmonary blood flow as a function of pulmonary artery pressure. It is assumed that pulmonary vein pressure is constant at 8 mmHg. The pink line represents the relationship for a system of tubes that does not "give" with increasing transmural pressure.

The importance of this passive/compliant pressure-flow relationship is best appreciated by considering what happens during exercise. The cardiac output can increase 4 or 5 fold with only a moderate increase in mean pulmonary artery pressure. For example, using Figure 1, an increase of mean pulmonary artery pressure of only 50% (from 14 to 21 mmHg) is consistent with a 3-fold increase in cardiac output. The key: distension of resistance vessels and recruitment of more capillaries.

Increases in pulmonary <u>vein</u> pressure also expand the pulmonary microcirculation and result in decreased resistance to flow. This effect is not as pronounced as that from increased pulmonary artery pressure, but it probably accounts for the fact that in left heart failure an increase in pulmonary artery pressure may be delayed and attenuated compared to the increase in left atrial and pulmonary vein pressure.

Effect of Lung Volume on PVR

As lung volume increases from residual volume on up, not only do alveoli expand but, to some degree, extra-alveolar arteries and veins also expand, which tends to decrease PVR. But also as lung volume increases and the alveoli expand, the alveolar capillary networks are stretched lengthwise. This causes the capillaries to get skinnier and tends to increase PVR. The latter effect is especially prominent at lung volumes above FRC. The overall effect is biphasic and is shown in Figure 2. Minimum PVR occurs at roughly FRC.

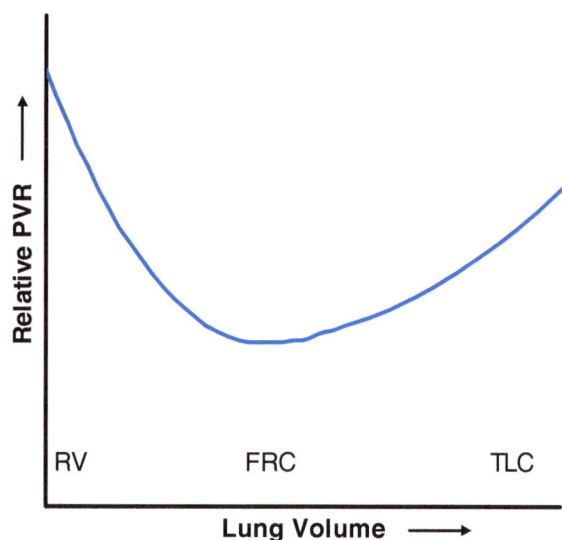

Figure 2. Pulmonary vascular resistance as a function of lung volume.

Thus, during a normal tidal inspiration, PVR increases. The physiological importance of this relationship is not clear, but it may contribute to the fact that during inspiration left ventricular stroke volume and, therefore, arterial systolic pressure decline a little.

Other Influences on PVR

Neural

The pulmonary vessels, including arterioles, are innervated by autonomic nerves, but rather sparsely, and the role of autonomic activity in regulating PVR is thought not to be important.

Endocrine (hormonal)

Circulating humoral agents such as angiotensin II do have effects on pulmonary smooth muscle, but again, their role is thought to be minimal.

Paracrine

A paracrine is a chemical that acts near its site of release. This is in contrast to a hormone that is carried in blood and acts some distance from its site of release. Some paracrines might be very important in regulating PVR. These include nitric oxide (NO) and endothelin 1. These will be mentioned when we discuss hypoxic vasoconstriction.

Part 2: Some Principles of Blood Flow in Pulmonary Capillaries

Topic 1: Capillary Recruitment

Pulmonary artery pressure minus pulmonary vein pressure is the overall driving force for pulmonary blood flow, and this is always positive. Nevertheless, there are ordinarily many capillaries with no flow. This is due to random variations in pressure drop along the resistance vessels. Sometimes the pressure drop is so much by the time individual capillaries are reached that they have no flow. They are still open, just not flowing. Even reverse flow sometimes occurs. With greater pulmonary artery pressure, these capillaries may start flowing, *i.e.* they can be recruited. Flow in some capillaries may be stopped by red cell rouleaux or perhaps by white cells that have a hard time getting through. Increased driving pressure may break up the rouleaux or force the white cells through, again recruiting more capillaries.

Topic 2: Capillary Squeeze

The axial pressure difference (upstream minus downstream) is the force that drives flow through any tube. However, if the tube is collapsible the transmural pressure difference (inside minus outside) can play an important role. If outside pressure exceeds inside pressure the tube will be squeezed. Its lumen might be completely obliterated if the negative transmural pressure is great enough to overcome the structural forces in the tube wall that try to keep it round. In this case there would be no flow. These structural forces in capillaries are very weak, and the no-flow state due to squeeze can actually happen in alveolar capillaries if alveolar air pressure becomes greater than capillary blood pressure. Ordinarily, complete capillary occlusion does not happen anywhere in the lungs unless alveolar pressure is increased by positive pressure ventilation, or the capillary blood pressure is severely decreased because of hypovolemia.

A more common situation in the lungs is partial squeeze. The transmural pressure (blood minus alveolar) can become negative enough to reduce the capillary diameter but not completely occlude it. The result is an increase in resistance to flow.

Topic 3: Capillary Flutter

If transmural pressure becomes just negative enough to occlude a capillary, flow stops. When flow stops there is no longer a pressure drop along the precapillary resistance vessels and, therefore, pressure rises in the capillary. The capillary then opens and flow resumes. Then a pressure drop along the precapillary resistance vessels develops again, the capillary collapses, and flow stops, *etc*. Flow flutters. The effective resistance to flow has increased. Now, flow is not much determined by axial pressure difference, but mainly by transmural pressure difference.

Flutter flow has often been called a vascular waterfall since the flow over a waterfall is not influenced by downstream pressure or height of the fall. The analogy is not good, however, since flow over a waterfall has nothing to do with transmural pressure and it doesn't flutter.

Topic 4: Intermittent Flow Due to Cardiac and Breathing Cycles

Flutter flow is, of course, intermittent flow. But there is a simpler cause of intermittent flow. During the cardiac cycle pulmonary artery pressure rises and falls. To a lesser extent, this is also true of the breathing cycle. Thus, some pulmonary capillaries might be compressed (increased resistance) during diastole and rounded back up during systole. Pulmonary artery pressure drops a little during inspiration and comes back up during expiration; this cycle can have a minor effect on capillary transmural pressure and, therefore, on resistance to flow.

Part 3: Regional Variations in Blood Flow

Topic 1: The Blood Flow Gradient from Base to Apex

The regional distribution of alveolar ventilation was described in Chapter 3. Briefly, in an upright person at FRC, alveoli near the top of the lungs (apex) are already fairly well inflated so during inspiration they do not inflate much more. Alveoli near the base of the lungs are somewhat deflated at FRC and during inspiration they inflate a lot. Thus there is a gradient in alveolar ventilation, increasing from apex to base. The mechanism of this gradient is not entirely clear. It is influenced by gravity but the basic structure of the lungs may also be important.

There is a similar gradient for alveolar blood flow, increasing from apex to base. The gradient for blood flow is considerably more pronounced than that for alveolar ventilation. Thus, the ratio of ventilation to perfusion progressively decreases from apex to base of the lungs. This ratio is called the $\dot{V}/\dot{Q}$ ratio. $\dot{V}$ is the rate of air flow and $\dot{Q}$ is the rate of blood flow. The $\dot{V}/\dot{Q}$ ratio for the whole lung is normally a little over 0.8 (*e.g.*: if alveolar ventilation = 4.5 L/min and cardiac output = 5.5 L/min).

The perfusion gradient has traditionally been explained by gravity but it now appears that the basic anatomy of the pulmonary circulation may also be important. Here are the explanations for the blood flow gradient:

Explanation Based on Gravity

Distention and Recruitment:
In an upright person, arterial pressure increases from apex to base of the lungs. This is simply a hydrostatic effect: pressure in a continuous column of fluid depends on height. The result is that there is more distension of vessels and recruitment of capillaries leading to less resistance to flow as the lungs are descended.

Collapse and Intermittent Flow:
Since capillary pressure is greatest at the base of the lung (upright person) and progressively decreases toward the apex, the flow characteristics that are due to squeezing of capillaries, collapse and intermittent flow, are more likely to occur as the lung is ascended.

[Perhaps we should look at some numbers. Pulmonary artery pressure at mid-lung is normally about 24/9 mmHg. Near the apex (upright person) the pressures are less, roughly 12/-3 mmHg, and at the base they are more, about 36/21 mmHg due to hydrostatic effects. Alveolar pressure averages zero with small variations (usually less than 1 mmHg) during breathing.]

Explanation Based on Anatomy
The importance of gravity for determining the apex-to-base perfusion gradient was based on techniques with rather limited spatial resolution (mainly distribution of radioactive xenon). Newer methods with greater spatial resolution (mainly using labeled microspheres) have demonstrated that the basic structure of the pulmonary vascular system is important. The vessels near the base apparently branch in ways that reduce resistance more than those near the apex (more branches in parallel, larger branches).

The relative importance of gravity *vs.* structure is currently a highly controversial subject. The issue has been argued in *J. Applied Physiology,* Nov., 2007.

Consequences for O_2 Delivery to the Systemic Circulation

Consider the alveoli near the apex of the lungs in an upright person. These alveoli are relatively poorly ventilated. Consequently, they have a relatively low PO_2 and high PCO_2. Blood flowing past these alveoli is deficient in O_2 and rich in CO_2. High blood flow in these regions could lead to arterial hypoxemia and CO_2 retention. So it is good that blood flow is reduced in the apex.

On the other hand, since alveoli near the base of the lungs are especially well ventilated it is good that they have more blood flow than those near the apex. More oxygen delivery from basal alveoli ought to make up for less oxygen delivery from apical alveoli. But there is a catch. It is true that more O_2 is delivered per unit time from basal alveoli than from an equal number of apical alveoli, but it is delivered at a lower PO_2. This results from the fact that blood flow increases toward the base more than does ventilation. The result is a small reduction in arterial PO_2! Thus, arterial PO_2 is slightly decreased by reduced O_2 delivery from apical alveoli and also from delivery of blood with a reduced PO_2 from basal alveoli. This complex phenomenon will be more thoroughly explained in Chapters 9 and 10.

In 1964 the great pulmonary physiologist, John West, introduced the concept of zones in the lungs for the effect of gravity on blood flow. Zone 1 (toward the top): capillaries are susceptible to complete occlusion under some abnormal circumstances (pulmonary hypotension, alveolar positive pressure). Zone 2 (mid-lung) is normally susceptible to intermittent flow. Zone 3 (toward the base) is generally immune from these problems. Despite the term "zone", there are no anatomical demarcations, and which zone any particular part of the lung is in depends on the circumstances. For example, the entire lung is normally in zones 2 and 3, but the entire lung could be in zones 1 and 2 with positive pressure breathing. Nevertheless, the zone concept is classic and always taught. I personally think it has added confusion with little reward in understanding. But you probably need to know about it.

Part 4: Hypoxic Vasoconstriction

Topic 1: General

So far we have presented the pulmonary circulation as a system that responds passively to pressure changes and have downgraded the importance of active responses to neural and humoral stimuli. However, there is a very important exception. Low alveolar PO_2 results in arteriolar constriction and reduced blood flow. This phenomenon is known as hypoxic pulmonary vasoconstriction (HPV). The result is that poorly ventilated alveoli get less blood flow. This is good. Why waste blood flow on laggard alveoli? Divert it to alveoli that can do more for the cause – arterialization of the blood. Of course this traffic control is more important than simply not wasting blood flow, since blood equilibrating with low PO_2 alveoli will send low PO_2 blood to the systemic circulation and if this occurred a lot, it could result in arterial hypoxemia.

Curiously, HPV is far more sensitive to low PO_2 in alveolar air than to low PO_2 in blood. In fact, changes in blood PO_2 have almost no effect.

However, blood pH does have an effect. Low blood pH increases the sensitivity of HPV to low alveolar PO_2.

Topic 2: The Mechanism of Hypoxic Pulmonary Vasoconstriction

Although HPV was discovered in 1946 our knowledge of the mechanism is still sketchy. Nerves are definitely not involved; HPV occurs in transplanted lungs. It is thought that the signal (low P_AO_2) may act directly on vascular smooth muscle. Currently, reactive oxygen species (ROS) are getting a lot of attention; they may act to close a redox-sensitive voltage-gated potassium channel (K_V) in smooth muscle. When this channel closes, the smooth muscle membrane depolarizes, leading to contraction. Decreased nitric oxide (NO) and increased endothelin-1 from endothelium may also be involved. The possibility that decreased NO is important in HPV has led to its use in ICUs to treat hypoxemia.

Part 5: Fluid Balance among Blood, Interstitial Space, and Alveoli

Part 1: Basic Principles

Filtration of fluid across any capillary endothelium is driven by the resultant of four pressures, often called the Starling forces (*e.g.* see Baker's *Cardiovascular Physiology, 3rd Ed.*, p. 173). The net filtration pressure is given by

$$P_{net} = (P_c - P_i) - \sigma\,(\pi_c - \pi_i)$$

P_{net} = net filtration pressure
P_c = capillary hydrostatic pressure
P_i = interstitial hydrostatic pressure
π_c = capillary oncotic pressure (due to plasma proteins)
π_i = interstitial oncotic pressure (due to interstitial proteins and glycosaminoglycans)
σ = the reflection coefficient

The reflection coefficient is a correction factor that accounts for the fact that the effective oncotic pressure difference is often less than would be calculated from the protein concentrations. This happens when the endothelium is permeable to albumin and perhaps to other proteins. The reflection coefficient for pulmonary capillaries is normally close to 0.7. It can decrease with damage to the endothelium.

If net filtration pressure is positive, there is net fluid flux out of capillaries. Ordinarily, P_{net} is slightly positive and the resulting net fluid flux drains away in lymph with no accumulation in the interstitium.

The values for interstitial hydrostatic pressure and interstitial oncotic pressure are not known with any accuracy, so actual calculations of P_{net} cannot be made and are not really necessary. The principles expressed in the above fluid balance equation, however, are very important in understanding pulmonary edema (see below). Briefly, if P_c is too high, fluid moves into the interstitial spaces faster than it can be carried off in lymph and the interstitial spaces get water-logged. The same is true if π_c is too low, if P_i is too low, if π_i is too high, or if σ is too low. Any of these conditions can lead to interstitial edema. Build-up of interstitial edema fluid is somewhat self-limiting since as it occurs interstitial oncotic pressure is reduced and interstitial hydrostatic pressure is increased, and

eventually a new balance of Starling forces might be attained.

Topic 2: The Role of Interfacial Tension

Alveoli are separated from each other by the alveolar septae. Because of surface tension, the alveoli are constantly trying to get smaller and more spherical. Surface forces pull in opposite directions on each septum, thereby reducing interstitial hydrostatic pressure, and pulling water into the interstitial spaces from blood. Because the air-water interface in each alveolus is constantly trying to get smaller and more spherical, water is sucked into it from the interstitial space. The least spherical locations in the alveolus are at the septal corners. As they try to "round out", water is preferentially drawn into them.

Topic 3: Active Fluid Reabsorption

In addition to secreting pulmonary surfactant, alveolar type II cells actively transport Na^+ out of alveolar fluid into interstitial spaces with Cl^- and water moving with the Na^+, electrically and osmotically respectively. This helps keep alveoli dry and is normally quite effective. The rate that water enters alveoli because of surface forces is matched by the rate it is pumped back out.

Topic 2: The Role of Pulmonary Surfactant

This balance would not be possible without pulmonary surfactant (see Chapter 3). Pulmonary surfactant is extremely important for keeping the lungs dry (*i.e.* preventing pulmonary edema) since it greatly reduces the air-septal interfacial tension and, therefore, reduces the rate at which water is sucked from blood into interstitial spaces and from there into alveoli. Some experts think that preventing pulmonary edema is the most important function of pulmonary surfactant.

Topic 3: Pulmonary Edema

Interstitial Edema: As explained above, if the Starling forces are out of balance, the interstitial spaces can swell. This is called interstitial edema. It can also be caused by inadequate lymphatic drainage. Pure interstitial edema can actually be difficult to detect, but is sometimes seen as "bronchiolar cuffing" on radiographs.

Alveolar Edema: Sometimes when the interstitial spaces are swollen, something happens to the alveolar epithelium that allows fluid to pour out of the interstitial spaces into the alveoli, overwhelming the ability of the type II pneumocytes to pump it back out. This occurs alveolus by alveolus and essentially fills each one with fluid so it cannot be ventilated. The blood flowing around such a fluid-filled alveolus exchanges no O_2 or CO_2 and is simply shunted toward the pulmonary veins. The result is arterial hypoxemia. Shunting will be discussed in Chapters 9 and 10.

Just what happens to the alveolar epithelium that suddenly allows flow into the alveolus is not understood. We can simply put it in the category of "damage". It must be fairly severe damage since the alveolar edema fluid is often tinged with red cells.

Some Conditions that Can Lead to Pulmonary Edema
- Increased Capillary Hydrostatic Pressure (most common cause):
  - Left heart failure
  - Mitral Stenosis
  - Hypervolemia (fluid overload, usually iatrogenic from too much IV infusion)
- Decreased Plasma Oncotic Pressure (not often a primary cause of pulmonary edema, but it can exaggerate the effects of other causes)
  - Renal disease
  - Liver disease
  - Protein malnutrition
  - Hemodilution (due to fluid overload)
- Increased Capillary Permeability to Proteins (decreased σ)
  - Acute (adult) respiratory distress syndrome (ARDS)
  - Endotoxins (during sepsis)
  - Pneumonia
  - Oxygen toxicity
  - Inhaled toxins
- Lymphatic Insufficiency
  - Tumors
  - Interstitial fibrosis

Part 6: The Bronchial Circulation

The bronchial arteries arise variably, mainly from the aortic arch and thoracic aorta, and supply the bronchial tree and surrounding structures with oxygenated blood down to the level of the terminal bronchioles. More distal regions (respiratory bronchioles, alveolar ducts, alveolar sacs, and alveoli) get their oxygen from alveolar air. The bronchial circulation accounts for as much as 2% of the cardiac output.

Much bronchial venous blood, especially from higher order bronchi, enters bronchial veins and eventually returns to the right atrium. However, and this is the interesting part, at least half of the bronchial blood, especially from the more distal bronchi and bronchioles, returns to the left atrium via the pulmonary veins. This is made possible by profuse anastomoses between the small bronchial and pulmonary veins. There are even anastomoses between the bronchial and pulmonary systems at the level of capillaries and arterioles. The reason this is so interesting is that this venous blood from the bronchial circulation mixes with arterialized blood from the pulmonary circulation and slightly dilutes it – a process called venous admixture. Venous admixture from the bronchial circulation contributes to the fact that the PO_2 in systemic arterial blood is never quite as high as it is in alveolar air.

Part 7: Actions of the Lungs on Circulating Substances

The lungs receive the entire right ventricular output and the pulmonary endothelial surface area is immense. Thus the pulmonary endothelium is ideally situated to process substances in blood plasma, and it does. The following table lists some of the more important examples.

Table 2

Substance	Effect	Process
Angiotensin II	Produced from angiotensin I	Angiotensin converting enzyme (ACE)
Bradykinin	About 80% inactivated	Angiotensin converting enzyme (ACE)
Serotonin	Almost all removed	Uptake by endocytosis
Norepinephrine	About 30% removed (but no removal of epinephrine)	Uptake by endocytosis
Prostaglandins E_1, E_2, and F_{2a}	Almost all removed (but no removal of A_1, A_2, and I_2)	Uptake by endocytosis
Leukotrienes	Almost all removed	Uptake by endocytosis

Filtering

The lungs filter out junk circulating in the blood. The junk may include small clots, air bubbles, fat cells, loose cancer cells, clumped red cells, clumped platelets, etc. The lungs can handle this stuff better than most vascular beds since they have a great deal of capillary reserve, at least at rest. If some capillaries get plugged, others can be recruited. If some of this junk made it to the brain, stroke could occur, and plugging of small coronaries could also be disastrous. So filtration is an important function of the pulmonary circulation.

Particles trapped in pulmonary capillaries are eventually removed by macrophages or by lytic enzymes in the endothelium.

Part 9: What Can Go Wrong?

Pulmonary Edema
Pulmonary Embolism
Pulmonary Hypertension

Chapter 6

Transfer of O_2 and CO_2 between Alveolar Air and Blood

Part 1: A Little Anatomy
Part 2: Equilibration of O_2 and CO_2 across the Alveolar-Capillary Membrane
Part 3: What Can Go Wrong?

Part 1: A Little Anatomy

Topic 1: The Alveolar Septae

Figure 1

Oxygen moves from alveolar air to blood and on into red blood cells where most of it binds to hemoglobin. Carbon dioxide moves from blood to alveolar air. These processes are facilitated by a very close juxtaposition of the alveoli and capillaries.

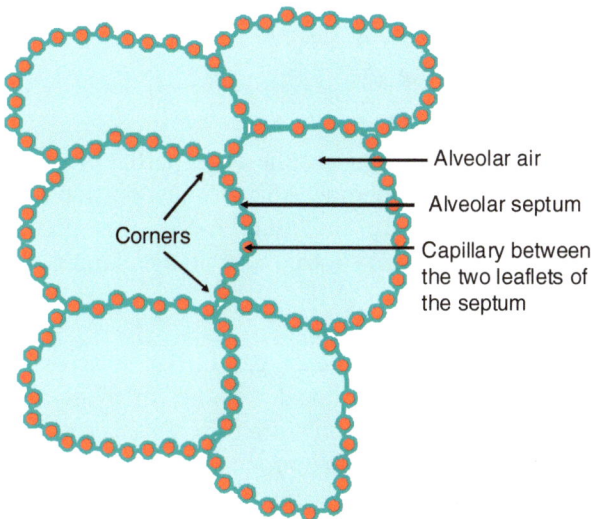

Figure 1. Diagram of a few adjacent alveoli in cross-section. The septae consist of the joined walls of adjacent alveoli. The areas where septae converge are called corners Capillaries course within the septum between adjacent alveolar walls. Single capillary networks may continue over more than one alveolus. The point of this diagram is to emphasize that much of each alveolar wall directly overlies a capillary. Alveolar capillary diameter is roughly 8-10 μm. Alveolar diameter averages about 100 μm.

Alveolar septae are the joined walls of adjacent alveoli. The capillaries are located within the alveolar septae, bulging between the wall of one alveolus and that of its neighbor. There are so many of these capillaries (due to profuse branching and anastomosis) that each alveolus is covered by a dense plexus of vascular capillaries. Figure 1 is a crude diagram to illustrate that a large fraction of each alveolar surface is in intimate contact with capillaries. Also see Figure 6 in Chapter 1.

Topic 2: The Alveolar-Capillary Membrane

Figure 2

The tissue that separates alveolar air from blood plasma consists of the alveolar epithelium (mostly type I pneumocytes) and the capillary endothelium with some basement membrane in between. In addition, on the inner surface of the alveoli there is a thin aqueous layer with surfactant at the air-water interface. These structures are diagrammed in Figure 2. Also see Figure 4 in Chapter 1. The entire complex is very thin, less than 0.5 μm except where there are epithelial or endothelial nuclei, or type II pneumocytes. It is important that this layer is thin so that diffusion distances are short.

The respiratory gases must move fast enough across the alveolar-capillary membrane to achieve equilibrium between air and blood within the time it takes for blood to flow through the capillaries, which is roughly 0.75 seconds. Long ago (1900 or so) there was controversy about the mechanism of gas movement across this complex membrane. Some prominent physiologists thought that active transport was involved, or as they called it then, "vital activity". Eventually, simple diffusion was established as the mechanism of respiratory gas transport across the alveolar-capillary membrane.

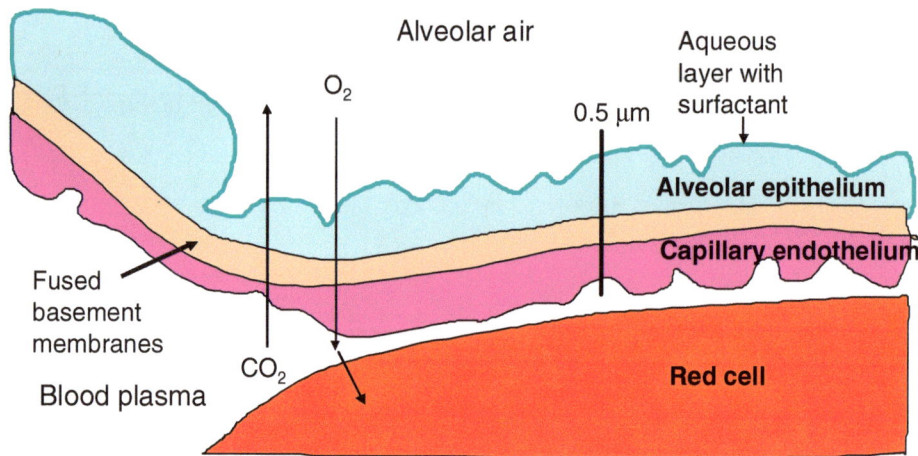

Figure 2. This diagram is redrawn (for simplicity) from an EM in *Wheater's Functional Histology*. Alveolar air is separated from blood plasma by alveolar epithelium, capillary endothelium, and their fused basement membranes. The diffusion distance is very short compared to the diameter of a red cell.

Part 2: Equilibration of O_2 and CO_2 across the Alveolar-Capillary Membrane

Topic 1: Diffusion

Some Principles

Fick's Law of diffusion as modified for diffusion across a membrane is:

$$Rate = A \cdot D_m \frac{C_1 - C_2}{w}$$

- Rate = the net rate of diffusion from side 1 to side 2 of the membrane
- A = area of the membrane
- D_m = the diffusion coefficient in the membrane
- w = thickness of the membrane
- C_1 and C_2 are concentrations of the diffusing substance on the two sides of the membrane (just within the membrane)

The concentration of a dissolved gas is directly proportional to its partial pressure, P.

$$C = s \times P$$

This is Henry's Law. The proportionality constant, s, is the solubility of the gas in the membrane.

Thus, Fick's Law for gas diffusion across a membrane becomes:

$$Rate = A \cdot D_m \cdot s \cdot \frac{P_1 - P_2}{w}$$

Assuming that the gas has the same partial pressure just inside the membrane as it does just outside (*i.e.* is equilibrated at the interfaces), the partial pressures in Equation 1 are those in alveolar air and in blood.

So we see that the rate of gas diffusion across a membrane is proportional to the area of the membrane, the partial pressure difference across the membrane, the diffusion coefficient in the membrane, and the solubility in the membrane; and is inversely proportional to the thickness of the membrane. Diffusion continues until $P_1 = P_2$ and then net diffusion stops.

[Note: The diffusion coefficient for a gas diffusing in the gaseous phase is inversely proportional to the square root of the molecular weight of the gas. This is Graham's Law and can be derived from the kinetic molecular theory of ideal gases. Graham's Law is reasonably accurate in alveolar air. Graham's Law is <u>not true</u> for dissolved gases diffusing in aqueous media or in membranes, contrary to what is stated in many textbooks of pulmonary physiology.]

Relative Rates of O_2 and CO_2 Diffusion across the Alveolar-Capillary Membrane

The alveolar-capillary wall is often conceptualized as a thin <u>aqueous</u> layer separating alveolar air from blood. Of course, this is not really true; there are also cell membranes. However, O_2 and CO_2 are lipid soluble enough to diffuse through cell membranes quite rapidly and the assumption of an aqueous layer is probably alright. The solubility of CO_2 in water is about 24-fold greater than that of O_2. On the other hand, D_m for CO_2 through an aqueous layer is a little less than that for O_2. The end result is that the permeability of the alveolar-capillary membrane for CO_2 is about 20-fold greater than for O_2.

Topic 2: There is Also Chemistry

There is, however, more to the process of gas exchange than diffusion across the alveolar-capillary membrane. Nearly all of the O_2 that enters blood plasma diffuses on into the red cells and then binds to hemoglobin. These processes take a finite amount of time, roughly as much time as it takes to diffuse from alveolar air to blood plasma. O_2 diffusion continues until hemoglobin is nearly saturated with O_2. Only then can PO_2 in plasma reach its final value, equal to alveolar PO_2.

CO_2 is mostly carried in blood plasma as bicarbonate. Plasma bicarbonate must move into red cells where it is converted to CO_2 and water, a reaction catalyzed by carbonic anhydrase. Then CO_2 must diffuse out of red cells before it can diffuse on into alveoli. Again, these chemical processes importantly influence the rates of the overall transfer process for CO_2.

Details of how O_2 and CO_2 are carried in blood and their chemical reactions will be discussed in Chapters 7 and 8.

Topic 3: Rates of Equilibration

Normal Person at Rest
Figure 3

Figure 3 shows the time line for capillary PO_2 and PCO_2 from start to finish along the alveolar-capillary interface for a single capillary plexus.

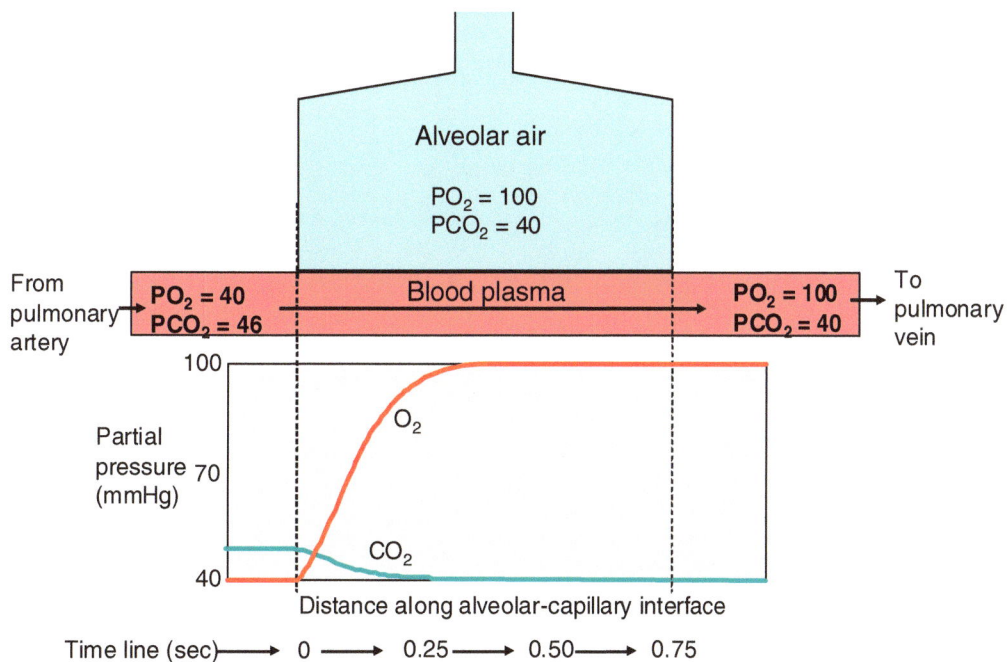

Figure 3. Time line for equilibration of O_2 and CO_2 along the alveolar-capillary membrane. At rest, O_2 is essentially equilibrated within about ¼ sec, or about one-third of the capillary length. It is less clear how long it takes for CO_2 to equilibrate, but it is said to be about the same as for O_2.

Normally, at rest, both O_2 and CO_2 equilibrate between alveolar air and blood plasma over the first third of the capillary. This takes about 0.25 seconds. The rate of equilibration, surprisingly, seems to be no faster for CO_2 than it is for O_2 even though CO_2 diffuses much faster. This behavior is partly explained by the fact that the initial partial pressure difference is about 10 times greater for O_2 than it is for CO_2. But even after taking this into account, one would think that the initial rate of equilibration for CO_2 would be about twice that for O_2.

Normal Person during Exercise

Cardiac output increases during exercise and, therefore, pulmonary blood flow increases. A portion of this increase is carried by newly recruited alveolar capillaries that open under an increase in pulmonary arterial pressure. Some is handled by passive dilation of capillaries caused by increased capillary pressure. But in addition to these passive compensations, the velocity of blood flow through alveolar capillaries increases. In strenuous exercise, velocity may increase 2 or 3 fold and the transit time may decrease from ¾ sec to ¼ sec. This is still enough time for both O_2 and CO_2 to equilibrate between alveolar air and blood plasma, barely enough time for O_2, but plenty of time for CO_2.

Person with Thickened Alveolar-Capillary Membrane

Conditions that result in thickening of the alveolar-capillary membrane and, therefore, increase the length of the diffusion path include pulmonary interstitial edema, interstitial fibrosis, and alveolar edema. These conditions can lead to failure of O_2 equilibration, especially during exercise, with an increased A-a PO_2 gradient. Arterial hypoxemia can be a consequence. These conditions seldom lead to failure of CO_2 equilibration and $PaCO_2$ is usually the same as P_ACO_2.

Person with Decreased Alveolar Surface Area

Emphysema is a disease that causes deterioration of pulmonary connective tissue and results in small airway collapse due to failure of radial traction. It also results in breakdown of alveolar septae. Alveoli coalesce and total alveolar surface area decreases. The decrease in surface area slows net diffusion of O_2. This effect can be severe enough that O_2 equilibration fails, the A-a PO_2 gradient increases, and arterial hypoxemia results, especially

during exercise. Again, CO_2 equilibration is usually not compromised.

Topic 4: Insensitivity of CO_2 Equilibration to Changes in its Rate of Diffusion

Failure for alveolar capillary CO_2 to equilibrate with alveolar air almost never happens. Therefore, the PCO_2 in pulmonary veins and even in systemic arteries is usually the same as that in alveolar air. In other words, the A-a PCO_2 difference is generally zero. This is true even when the thickness of the alveolar-capillary membrane is increased as a result of interstitial pulmonary congestion or fibrosis. The only exception to this rule is when there is a significant amount of blood that flows from pulmonary artery to pulmonary veins without having a chance to equilibrate with air in ventilated alveoli. This is called a shunt and will be discussed in a later chapter.

On the other hand, as we have already seen, alveolar O_2 may fail to equilibrate with capillary blood in diseases that increase the length of the diffusion path or decrease the surface area. The result can be an abnormally large A-a O_2 gradient and arterial hypoxemia.

Topic 5: Role of Carbonic Anhydrase

The fact that CO_2 equilibration is almost immune to large changes in diffusion distance and surface area seems surprising. The usual textbook explanation is that equilibrium is always attained because CO_2 diffuses so fast. But there are problems with this simple explanation. For example, inhibition of carbonic anhydrase with drugs such as acetazolamide reduce the rate of CO_2 transfer and produce an appreciable A-a PCO_2 difference. The result is respiratory acidosis.

In fact, the rate of CO_2 transfer across the alveolar-capillary membrane is not limited as much by diffusion as it is by generation of CO_2 in red blood cells by the carbonic anhydrase reaction. Therefore, changes in diffusion distance and area are not expected to change the rate of CO_2 transfer as much as they change the rate of O_2 transfer.

Besides the carbonic anhydrase in red blood cells there are several other isoforms of carbonic anhydrase in capillary endothelium and in alveolar epithelium. Some of these carbonic anhydrases are thought to facilitate CO_2 transfer, but the mechanisms are not understood.

Topic 6: Clinical Measurement of Lung Diffusing Capacity

The rate at which carbon monoxide (CO) diffuses out of alveolar air is often measured in order to test for possible diffusion impairment. A very low, innocuous concentration of CO is inhaled. In the single breath version of the technique, a vital capacity volume is inhaled; the breath is held for about 10 sec and then exhaled down to residual volume. CO concentrations are measured in inspired and expired alveolar air. There are more details, but the bottom line is that the rate of CO uptake into blood (in ml/min) can be determined. This value is then divided by the partial pressure of CO in alveolar air, P_ACO. [Arterial PCO is assumed to be essentially zero because CO rapidly and avidly binds to hemoglobin.] The result is usually called the diffusing capacity of the lung for CO, abbreviated, D_LCO. However, it is important to realize that the measured value for D_LCO is not only determined by the properties of the alveolar-capillary membrane (A, D_m, s, and w), but also by diffusion through blood plasma, the red cell membrane, and the hemoglobin-packed red cell interior. It is also influenced by the rate at which CO binds to hemoglobin and, consequently, it is influenced by hemoglobin concentration and pulmonary capillary blood volume. A more appropriate term for this measurement (used more in Europe) is transfer factor, but it looks like we are stuck with diffusing capacity.

Part 3: What Can Go Wrong?

Conditions that Decrease D_LCO

Thickening of the Alveolar-Capillary Membrane
        Interstitial or alveolar edema
        Interstitial or alveolar fibrosis
            Sarcoidosis
            Scleroderma

Decreased Surface Area
        Emphysema
        Tumors
        Low cardiac output
        Low pulmonary capillary blood volume

Decreased Uptake by Erythrocytes
        Anemia
        Low pulmonary capillary blood volume

Ventilation-Perfusion Mismatch (to be discussed in Chapter 9)

[This list is slightly modified from M.G. Levitsky, *Pulmonary Physiology, 6th Ed.*, McGraw-Hill, 2003.]

Chapter 7

Oxygen Transport from Lungs to Tissues

Part 1: Hemoglobin
Part 2: Oxygen-Hemoglobin Dissociation Curves
Part 3: Other Hemoglobins
Part 4: Advantages of Packaging Hemoglobin in Red Cells
Part 5: What Can Go Wrong?

Part 1: Hemoglobin

Topic 1: Structure of Hemoglobin

Figures 1, 2, and 3

Hemoglobin is a tetrameric protein having a molecular weight of about 68,000 Daltons. It is abbreviated Hb. Each of its four subunits consists of a globular polypeptide chain (called a globin) with an attached porphyrin group that contains Fe^{++} (ferrous iron). The porphyrin with iron is called a heme group. Two of the polypeptides are identical and are called α chains. The other two are also identical and are called β chains. The four subunits are stuck together by salt bridges, hydrogen bonds, and hydrophobic effects. A diagram of Hb is shown in Figure 1.

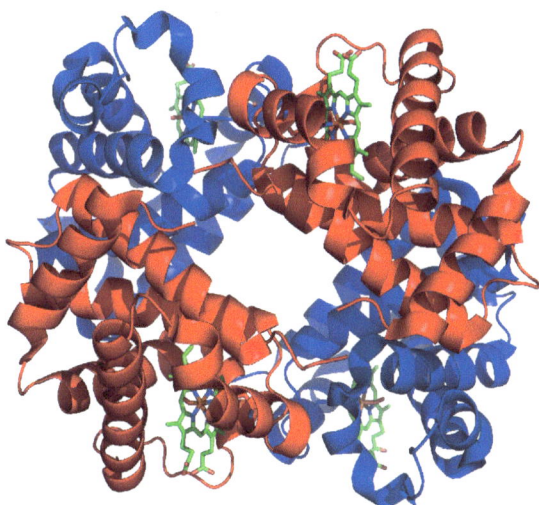

Figure 2. Deoxygenated hemoglobin. Hemes are in red. This image was constructed from the Protein Data Base (PDB) file 2dhb by S. Dutta and D.S. Goodsell. It was downloaded from www.pdb.org.

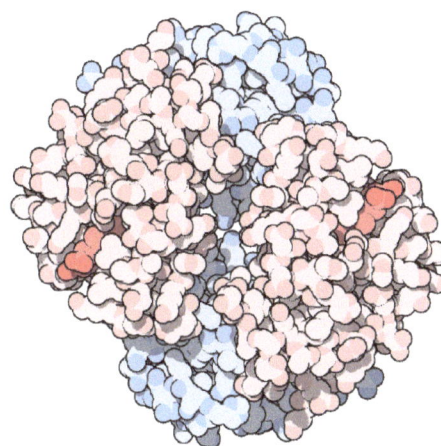

Figure 1. Ribbon diagram of hemoglobin. Globin chains are red and blue, heme groups are green. From the Protein Data Base, PDB ID: 1dgx. M. Paoli, *et al.*, J. Mol. Biol. 256:775-792, 1996.

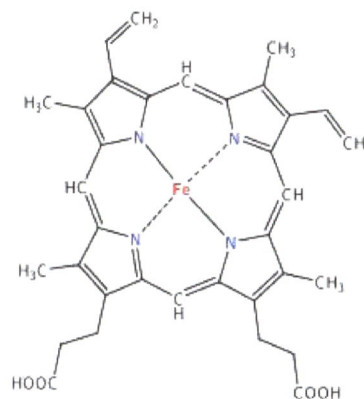

Figure 3. Heme group without O_2. The iron sticks up just a little out of the porphyrin plane. From Wikimedia Commons.

Topic 2: Some Chemistry of Hemoglobin

Porphyrin is constructed from four pyrrole groups. The ferrous iron of heme is coordinated with all four pyrrole groups and to the associated globin chain *via* a histidine. The ferrous iron can also bind O_2. Since there are four subunits, Hb can bind as many as four oxygens. When Hb has four bound oxygens, it is called oxyhemoglobin, abbreviated HbO_2. When Hb has no bound O_2 it is called deoxyhemoglobin. Deoxyhemoglobin is sometimes referred to as reduced hemoglobin, although this terminology is disappearing. The heme groups absorb visible light at wavelengths that result in Hb having a red color when O_2 is bound to all four hemes, giving way to a blue or purple color as O_2 unbinds. When O_2 binds to Fe^{++} the iron is not oxidized to Fe^{+++} (ferric iron), although it would be oxidized if the iron were not attached to porphyrin and a globin.

DeoxyHb is said to be in a tense (T) conformation, indicating that there is considerable strain on many of the bonds. Each heme group is lodged in a "pocket" near the surface of its globin chain. Fe^{++} is attached to globin via a histidine group and this is one of the bonds that is under strain. In the T state, these O_2 binding pockets are guarded by amino acid side chains and it is difficult for O_2 to enter. Consequently, initial binding of O_2 is rather slow. However, as soon as one O_2 molecule binds to any one of the four Fe^{++}s, the entire Hb molecule rearranges to the so-called relaxed (R) conformation. In the R conformation, O_2 can much more readily gain access to the binding pockets and to Fe^{++}. Therefore, as soon as one Fe^{++} successfully binds an O_2, the other three Fe^{++}s almost instantaneously bind O_2s. This is a famous example of positive cooperativity (perhaps the most famous in biochemistry).

Thus, Hb tends to have either zero or four attached oxygens. Intermediates (with 2 or 3 oxygens exist but do not last long and, therefore, are relatively rare.

Figure 4

The Fe^{++} of deoxygenated heme extends out a little from the flat plane of porphyrin. This is the only way it can fit. But, when one O_2 binds to one of the four Fe^{++}s of Hb the situation changes; this oxygenated Fe^{++} now moves into the porphyrin plane and pulls on its attached histidine, which in turn tugs on its globin . It is this tug that triggers the T to R conformational change in the entire tetrameric protein. This trigger is illustrated in Figure 4.

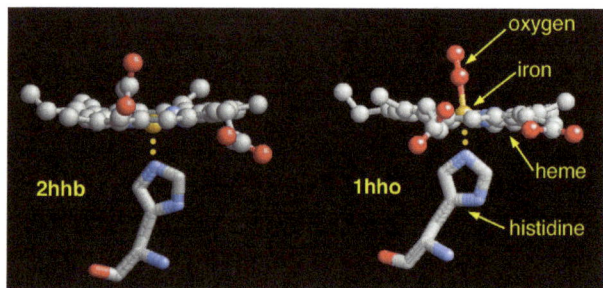

Figure 4. The trigger for the T to R transformation. Deoxygenated heme on the left, oxygenated heme on the right. Note that when O_2 binds, the histidine is pulled toward the heme thereby tugging on its globin (not shown here). The codes 2hhb and 1hho refer to the Protein Data Base (PDB) identification numbers. The image above was constructed from these data files by S. Dutta and D.S. Goodsell. It was downloaded from www.pdb.org.

Part 2: Hb-O₂ Dissociation Curves

Topic 1: The Basic Curve

Figure 5
As the partial pressure of O_2 in blood increases, the amount of O_2 bound to Hb increases up to a maximum of 1.34 ml of O_2/g of Hb. The curve relating bound O_2 to PO_2 is called the Hb-O_2 binding curve, equilibrium curve, or usually dissociation curve. The Hb-O_2 dissociation curve is S-shaped as shown in Figure 5.

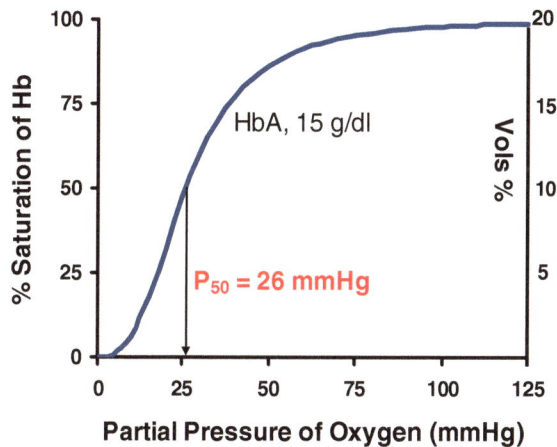

Figure 5. The Hb-O_2 dissociation curve. This is for human adult Hb (called HbA) at 37° C, $PCO_2 = 40$ mmHg, and pH = 7.4. Left ordinate is % saturation. Right ordinate is volume of O_2 carried by hemoglobin in 100 ml of blood, assuming 15.0 grams of Hb/100 ml; this is often called vols%. P_{50} is the partial pressure of O_2 required to reach 50% saturation.

The S shape of the Hb-O_2 dissociation curve is determined by two factors:
1. At first, binding of O_2 is difficult, but after a Hb molecule binds a single O_2 molecule, subsequent binding becomes much easier. It is this positive cooperativity (explained above) that causes the up-swoop of the curve.
2. However, the number of binding sites is limited and eventually, after most of the Fe^{++} sites are occupied by O_2, further binding levels off as saturation is approached.

The amount of O_2 binding can be expressed in two ways: % saturation or vols%. Often, both values are shown. As explained above, when Hb is 100% saturated with O_2, it has about 20 vols% O_2 (when blood contains 15 g% Hb).

Topic 2: The P_{50}

The P_{50} is the PO_2 at which Hb is 50% saturated with O_2, and is the usual way to express affinity. An increase in the P_{50} means that a higher PO_2 is necessary to reach 50% saturation, in other words the affinity for O_2 has decreased.

Remember:
A reduction in the P_{50} means that affinity for O_2 has increased. An increase in P_{50} means that affinity for O_2 has decreased. P_{50} is analogous to the Michaelis constant, K_M, in enzyme kinetics: a decrease in affinity of substrate for enzyme is indicated by an increase in K_M.

Topic 3: O₂ Carrying Capacity of Blood

One gram of Hb can bind as much as 1.34 ml of O_2. The normal concentration of Hb in blood is 15 g/100 ml). Therefore, 100 ml of blood can normally contain a maximum of 15 x 1.34 = 20.1 ml of O_2 bound to hemoglobin. At a normal arterial PO_2 of 100 mmHg, Hb is nearly 100% saturated with O_2 and actually does carry almost 20 ml of O_2 per 100 ml of blood. Percent saturation of Hb with O_2 is designated SaO_2 in arterial blood and SvO_2 in venous blood.

The solubility coefficient of O_2 in blood plasma at 37° C is about 0.003 ml/dl/mmHg. So at an arterial PO_2 of 100 mmHg, 100 ml of blood carries about 0.3 ml of physically dissolved O_2. This is a very small amount of O_2 compared to that carried by Hb and would be totally insufficient to keep up with O_2 demand. Hemoglobin is essential.

Topic 3: Loading of O₂ in the Lungs and Unloading in the Tissues

Loading of O₂ in the Lungs
The PO_2 in mixed venous blood (pulmonary artery) is about 40 mmHg in a normal person at rest, which means an SaO_2 of about 75%. Blood leaving the alveoli normally has a PO_2 of about 100 mmHg. It is obvious from Figure 5 that this is sufficient for nearly complete saturation of Hb with O_2.

Breathing 100% O_2 raises the PaO_2 much higher but results in only a minute increase in O_2 carried by

Hb. The utility of breathing 100% O_2 during athletic endeavors, therefore, has been questioned.

Above about 75 mmHg the curve is relatively flat. For example, at a PO_2 of 75 mmHg, Hb is still 95% saturated. Thus, there is a large safety factor for oxygen loading in the lungs. PaO_2 can drop quite a lot without harmful results. The clinical message is that pulmonary disorders that result in poor alveolar ventilation or result in a fairly large A-a PO_2 gradient, may not have noticeable effects on O_2 delivery to tissues until they are relatively advanced.

Unloading of O_2 in the Tissues

Arterial blood entering systemic tissues has a PO_2 approaching 100 mmHg and an SaO_2 approaching 100%. Within systemic tissues, capillary PO_2 is only about 20-40 mmHg. In this range the Hb-O_2 dissociation curve is quite steep. Therefore, release of O_2 is very sensitive to decreased tissue PO_2, which happens during increased activity. The result of this happy circumstance is that Hb releases more O_2 as more O_2 is needed.

A Note on Systemic Shunting of O_2:
In systemic tissues, an appreciable amount of O_2 diffuses from small arteries to counterflowing small veins and never actually reaches the capillaries and venules where almost all O_2 delivery to metabolizing cells takes place. Because of this shunting of O_2, the PO_2 in blood leaving a tissue can be considerably higher than it is in the capillaries.

A Note on Cyanosis:
Deoxygenated Hb is blue, while oxygenated Hb is red. When blood contains more than about 5 g/dl deoxygenated Hb it becomes blue and the skin can look distinctly bluish. This is called <u>cyanosis</u>. With a normal concentration of Hb in blood of 15 g/dl, cyanosis appears when about one third of it is deoxygenated. According to Figure 5, this would happen at a PO_2 of roughly 35 mmHg.

Optional:
The Hb-O_2 dissociation curve is described by the following equation:

$$\% Sat = \frac{PO_2^n}{P_{50}^n + PO_2^n}$$

For the curve in Figure 5, $P_{50} = 26.0$ mmHg and $n = 2.8$

Topic 4: Factors that Change the P_{50}

As noted above, the steepness of the Hb-O_2 dissociation curve in metabolizing tissues assures that O_2 delivery increases as need increases. However, it gets even better than this – read on.

The Bohr Effect: Increased PCO_2 Causes Increased P_{50}
Figure 6
As oxidative metabolism increases, more CO_2 is generated and local tissue PCO_2 rises a little. This increases P_{50} (reduces affinity for O_2) and, therefore, more O_2 is unloaded from Hb. Get it? Increased local oxidative metabolism begets increased oxygen delivery. This effect of increased PCO_2 is called the Bohr Effect after Christian Bohr who discovered it in 1904 (incidentally he was the father of the famous atomic physicist, Neils Bohr).

The Bohr Effect is illustrated in Figure 6.

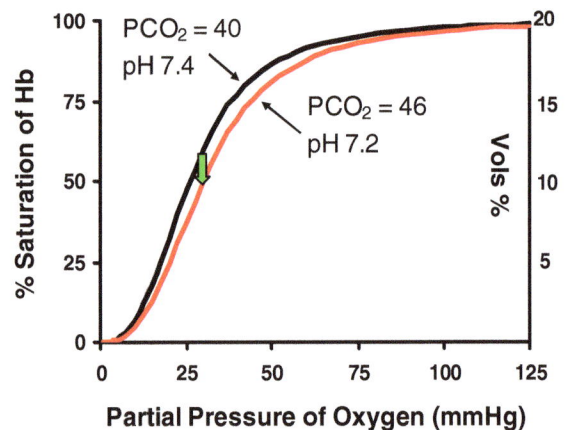

Figure 6. The Bohr Effect. Increased local PCO_2 causes decreased affinity of Hb for O_2 (*i.e.* increased P_{50}). Therefore, more O_2 is delivered to actively metabolizing tissue. [An increase in PCO_2 from 40 to 46 mmHg increases P_{50} from 26 to roughly 30 mmHg.]

An increase in local PCO_2 from 40 to 46 mmHg results in a decline in O_2 affinity, enough decline that at a PO_2 of 30 mmHg SaO_2 drops from 60% to 50% and appreciably more O_2 is delivered to the actively metabolizing tissue.

The Bohr Effect operates mainly *via* increased local acidity. CO_2 is quickly hydrated to carbonic acid (catalyzed by carbonic anhydrase) which immediately dissociates to hydrogen ions and bicarbonate. Here is the reaction:

$$CO_2 + H_2O \overset{ca}{\Leftrightarrow} H_2CO_3 \Leftrightarrow H^+ + HCO_3^-$$

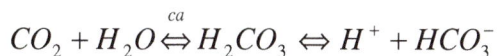

ca = carbonic anhydrase

This is an extremely important reaction. Increased generation of CO_2 in any local region causes this region to become a little more acidic (increased H^+ concentration, lower pH). The increased H^+ concentration titrates acid groups on globin, which results in an allosteric decrease in O_2 affinity.

Optional:
The mechanism of the Bohr Effect is interesting. Recall the T-to-R transformation of hemoglobin when it binds O_2. Binding to one heme greatly increases the affinity of the other three hemes for O_2. But another thing happens; a number of acid groups on globins ionize, releasing H^+. When, in actively metabolizing tissues, the H^+ concentration increases, release of H^+ from globin is partially reversed simply by mass action, and this tends to reverse the T-to-R transformation a little, causing some additional O_2 to be released from Hb and delivered to the tissues. In other words, the affinity between Hb and O_2 is reduced and P_{50} is increased.

An increase in PCO_2 is not the only thing that can elicit the Bohr Effect; it can also result from increased acidity due to lactic acid released from anaerobic metabolism.

Effect of Temperature
Increased local metabolic rate increases the temperature of the region. Increased temperature causes increased P_{50} and even more O_2 is delivered from Hb.

Effect of DPG
Red blood cells contain a high concentration of 2,3-diphosphoglycerate (called 2,3-DPG), which is a by-product of anaerobic glycolysis. DPG binds to globin of deoxygenated Hb, but is released upon oxygenation. Increased binding of DPG to deoxygenated Hb causes an increase in the P_{50} and

more O_2 is released from Hb and delivered to the tissue.

The amount of DPG bound to Hb depends on its concentration in red cells. Normally, the molar concentrations of Hb and DPG are about equal. DPG concentration gradually increases when inhaled PO_2 is low for a few days. This happens during acclimatization to high altitudes. The role of DPG in O_2 delivery is thought not to be for short-term adjustments, but rather for long-term adaptation to low ambient PO_2.

Optional:
As discussed above, the T-to-R transformation as O_2 binds to heme, results in increased affinity for O_2 (positive cooperativity) and increased acidic strength of various globin groups (release of H^+). It also results in less affinity for DPG. Increased steady concentration of DPG partially reverses the T-to-R transformation (by mass action) and causes reduced affinity for O_2.

Figure 7
This figure shows Hb-O_2 dissociation curves for normal and elevated concentrations of red cell DPG. It also shows the curve with no DPG. In the latter case the P_{50} is 1.0 (very high affinity).

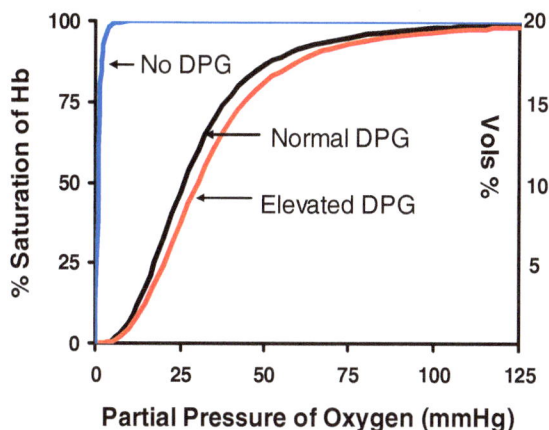

Figure 7. Effect of 2,3 DPG on the Hb-O_2 dissociation curve.

Part 3: Other Hemoglobins

Topic 1: Fetal Hemoglobin

Figure 8

Adult hemoglobin is appropriately called hemoglobin A (HbA). Fetal hemoglobin is slightly different and is called hemoglobin F (HbF). After birth, HbF is gradually replaced by HbA. The difference between the two is that HbA has two alpha globin chains and two beta chains ($\alpha2,\beta2$), while HbF has two alpha chains and two gamma chains ($\alpha2,\gamma2$). The switch from β to γ globins results in HbF having considerably less affinity for DPG and, therefore, a higher affinity for O_2. The P_{50} for HbF is only about 20 mmHg. This is illustrated in Figure 8.

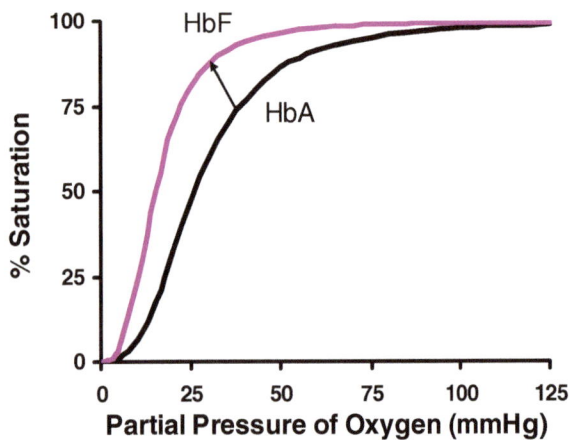

Figure 8. Fetal Hb has greater affinity for O_2 than adult Hb. Its P_{50} is much lower. The arrow indicates that when SaO_2 is 74% for maternal blood, it is 87% for fetal blood (see text).

As maternal blood flows through the placenta its PO_2 drops from roughly 95 to 38 mmHg. As fetal blood flows through the placenta its PO_2 rises from about 23 to 30 mmHg. It is apparent that O_2 does not fully equilibrate. This inadequacy is compensated by the higher affinity of HbF for O_2. At a PO_2 of 38 mmHg, maternal hemoglobin is about 74% saturated while at a PO_2 of only 30 mmHg, fetal hemoglobin is about 87% saturated. This is good for the fetus.

Topic 2: Methemoglobin

When the iron of Hb is oxidized to the ferric state (Fe^{+++}) it cannot bind oxygen. Oxidized Hb is called methemoglobin, abbreviated metHb. Various factors can convert Hb to metHb. One of the most interesting and perfectly normal examples is during the scavenging of nitric oxide by oxygenated hemoglobin. The NO is dioxygenated to NO_3^-, and in the process heme iron is oxidized resulting in metHb. However, red cells have an enzyme called <u>methemoglobin reductase</u> that quickly converts metHb back to regular Hb and all is well.

Other factors that can produce metHb include nitrites and various oxidative drugs. When metHb is excessive, the condition is called <u>methemoglobinemia</u>.

Topic 3: Carboxyhemoglobin and Carbon Monoxide Poisoning

Carbon monoxide (CO) binds to Hb with an affinity about 240 times that of O_2. The P_{50} for CO is only about 0.1 mmHg. O_2 and CO compete with each other for binding to hemoglobin Fe^{++}. If a Fe^{++} site has a CO attached, O_2 cannot attach. If blood Hb is 50% saturated with CO, then it can become, at most, 50% saturated with O_2. HbCO is usually called carboxyhemoglobin.

Acute CO poisoning can result from breathing fumes from incompletely burned carbon-based fuels. Culprits can be automobiles, malfunctioning space heaters, or fires. More insidious low-level CO poisoning can result from cigarette smoking. The result of CO poisoning can be depressed O_2 delivery to tissues, and when severe can lead to brain injury, and death.

In CO poisoning there is nothing wrong with alveolar ventilation or O_2 equilibration across the alveolar-capillary membrane. Therefore, there is nothing wrong with arterial PO_2. The problem is with arterial O_2 content. Curiously, the arterial chemoreceptors (Chapter 11) see nothing wrong since they are only sensitive to PO_2, not to O_2 content. Therefore, they fail to signal the respiratory centers in the brain to increase alveolar ventilation, which wouldn't do much good anyway. The point is that a person dying of CO poisoning might not seem to be in pulmonary distress until the muscles of inspiration give out due to hypoxia.

Figure 9

There is more to the problem than just decreased numbers of available O_2 binding sites on Hb. When one site is occupied by CO, the other three sites develop increased affinity for O_2 and, therefore, become reluctant to release O_2 in the tissues. In other words, the Hb-O_2 dissociation curve shifts to the left. It also becomes less sigmoid (more hyperbolic). So now, O_2 supply is jeopardized by decreased total O_2 in blood <u>and</u> by decreased release in the tissues. Figure 9 shows the combined effects of both problems on the Hb-O_2 dissociation curve.

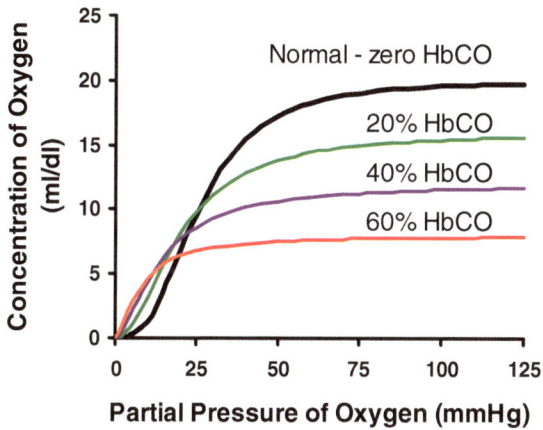

Figure 9. Hb-O_2 dissociation curves with various percentages of heme sites occupied by carbon monoxide.

Figure 10

This figure shows that as more heme sites are occupied by carbon monoxide, the amount of O_2 released in the tissues at 25 mmHg drops markedly. It also illustrates how much the change in affinity contributes to the problem.

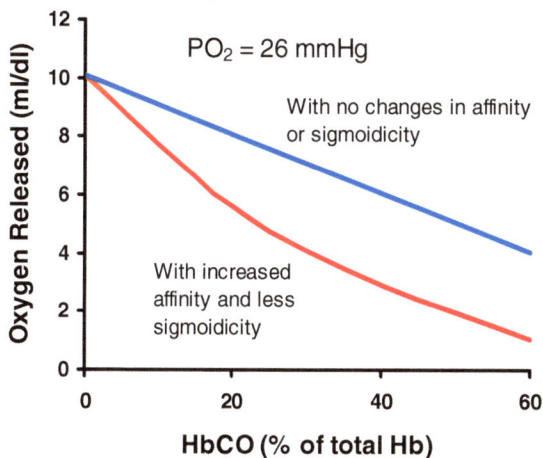

Figure 10. This figure shows how the percentage occupancy of Hb by CO affects the volume of O_2 released from Hb at a tissue PO_2 of 26 mmHg. The calculation assumes that the Hb was originally equilibrated at a PO_2 of 100 mmHg.

The affinity of fetal Hb for CO is about 10-15% higher than that for adult Hb. Therefore, CO poisoning of a pregnant woman can be even more dangerous for the fetus than for the mother.

The treatment for acute CO poisoning is simply breathing fresh air or preferably supplemental oxygen, and hope that O_2 will replace CO on Hb in time to avoid disaster.

Topic 4: Abnormal Hemoglobin Variants

Figure 11

Abnormal HbA variants number in the hundreds. Many of these hemoglobinopathies produce symptoms but most are extremely rare. The most common variant Hb is the one that causes sickle cell disease. This Hb is called HbS; it differs from normal HbA by only a single amino acid substitution in the β chains: valine is substituted for glutamic acid at position 6. Homozygotes for this mutation develop sickle cell disease while heterozygotes are carriers and are said to have sickle cell trait. HbS behaves like normal HbA as long as it is well oxygenated. But upon deoxygenation it can polymerize forming long, twisted, stiff fibers of HbS.

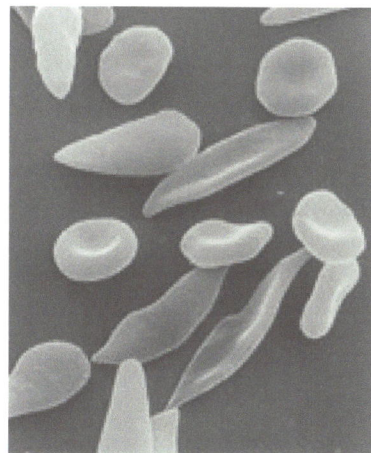

Figure 11. Red cells in sickle cell disease. Some cells are distorted by polymerized HbS.
Downloaded from Wikimedia Commons.

These HbS fibers can actually act like spikes that damage the red cell membrane. They frequently cause distortion of the red cell. This is shown in Figure 11. Sometimes the cells take on a crescent shape, giving the disease its name. Distorted red cells become fragile and, therefore, do not last as long as do normal red cells. Thus, anemia can develop. There also can be a major problem with these red cells clumping together and actually forming thrombi that occlude small arteries with resulting local ischemia and pain.

HbS is far more common in Sub-Saharan African people and their descendants than in most other groups. It is thought that it evolved due to the fact that it offers some protection against Malaria.

Topic 4: Myoglobin

Figure 12

Myoglobin is present at high concentration in striated muscle. It avidly binds O_2 with a P_{50} of only 1.0 mmHg. Myoglobin is monomeric. It consists of a globin polypeptide chain with an attached heme group. There is no positive cooperativity and, therefore, the dissociation curve is hyperbolic rather than S-shaped as seen in Figure 12.

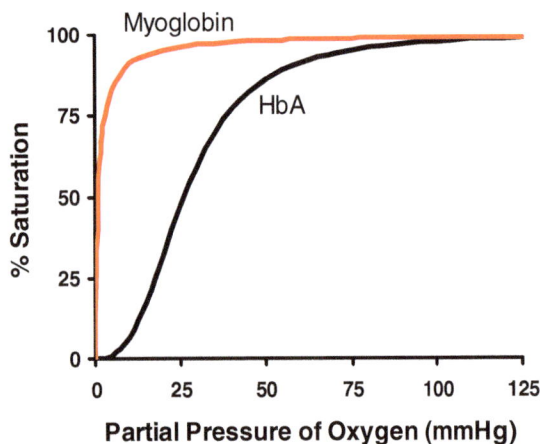

In resting skeletal muscle, myoglobin is more than 90% saturated. However, in maximally active skeletal muscle PO_2 drops so much that myoglobin saturation can go as low as 20%.

There are two functions of myoglobin within striated muscle cells. 1) Myoglobin stores O_2 which can then be used by muscle mitochondria in times of hypoxemia. 2) Myoglobin facilitates the diffusion of O_2 through muscle cytoplasm from the sarcolemma to mitochondria. The first function is important in diving mammals and birds, and they have especially high myoglobin concentrations. But for the rest of us the second function is thought to be far more important.

Figure 12. Myoglobin-O_2 dissociation curve compared to HbA-O_2 dissociation curve. The myoglobin curve is strongly left-shifted and is hyperbolic rather than sigmoid.

Part 4: Advantages of Packaging Hb in Red Cells

Topic: Why have red cells?

Prevention of Renal Loss of Hb
Free Hb tetramers tend to break down to monomers in plasma. Monomers are just small enough to be slightly filtered in the renal glomeruli and lost. Sequestering them in red cells prevents this.

Oncotic Pressure
If all the Hb packaged in red cells were dissolved in plasma, the protein osmotic pressure (oncotic pressure) of plasma would be far too high, and tissues would become dehydrated.

Viscosity
If all the Hb packaged in red cells were dissolved in plasma, the viscosity of plasma would increase about 3 or 4 fold and, therefore, peripheral resistance would markedly increase. Red cells increase the viscosity of blood in large vessels. At normal hematocrit, this effect is also about 4 fold. But as whole blood flows through the microcirculation, its viscosity decreases about to the level of plasma viscosity. This is called the Fahraeus-Lindqvist effect. It results from the combined effects of plug flow, the sigma effect, and reduced hematocrit, all of which are entirely dependent on red cells (see Baker's *Cardiovascular*

Physiology, 3rd Edition., p. 104-105).   The Fahraeus-Lindqvist effect is absolutely essential to keep total peripheral resistance low. Without red cells and with all the Hb dissolved in plasma, there would be no Fahraeus-Lindqvist effect and total peripheral resistance would be extremely high.

Nitric Oxide

It is essential that a low concentration of nitric oxide (NO) be present continuously in the vicinity of vascular smooth muscle in order to maintain low peripheral resistance.   Oxygenated heme avidly scavenges NO. It binds to Fe^{++} and is then rapidly converted to nitrate (NO_3^-) by a <u>dioxygenation</u> reaction.   The nitrate is then released and is harmless.

Some NO also binds to <u>deoxygenated</u> heme and is either converted to nitrite (NO_2^-) or is transferred to a cysteine residue on globin to form S-nitroso-hemoglobin.   The relative importance of these pathways is highly controversial. There is evidence that heme can convert NO_2^- back to NO in relatively hypoxic conditions and this may contribute to increased blood flow and O_2 delivery as needed. There is also evidence that S-nitroso-hemoglobin can release NO when PO_2 falls, further contributing to metabolic autoregulation.

If NO were scavenged too fast by Hb, total peripheral resistance would be too high. In fact, this is a serious problem in developing blood substitutes based on Hb derivatives. These are called hemoglobin-based oxygen carriers, HBOCs. Such blood substitutes dissolved in plasma may carry and release O_2 just fine, but they result in unacceptable increases in peripheral resistance, and so far have been disappointing for treating hypovolemia in spite of a tremendous amount of research effort and money.   Too much NO scavenging is thought to be a major problem. A relative deficit of the Fahraeus-Lindqvist effect may also be important since it requires the hemoglobin to be sequestered in red cells.

When Hb is sequestered in red cells, it scavenges NO more slowly than when it is dissolved in plasma, thereby allowing the vasodilatory effect of NO to be maintained at appropriate levels. It is not clear how this works. It has been proposed that there is actually a diffusion barrier around red cells that slows entry of NO.

Part 5: What Can Go Wrong?

Assuming alveolar ventilation and alveolar-capillary gas exchange are working properly, and there is adequate ambient O_2, there are only two general problems that compromise oxygen delivery to tissues: circulation problems and hemoglobin problems.

Circulation Problems
      Heart failure
      Increased resistance to flow
          Polycythemia
          Atherosclerosis
          Blood clots
          Tumors

Hemoglobin Problems
      Anemias
      Carbon monoxide poisoning
      Hemoglobinopathies, mainly sickle cell
          disease

Chapter 8

Transport of Carbon Dioxide from Tissues to Lungs

Part 1: Diffusion of CO_2 from Tissue Cells to Blood
Part 2: Paths Taken by CO_2 after Entering Blood
Part 3: Paths Taken by CO_2 in the Lungs
Part 4: The CO_2 Dissociation Curve

Part 1: Diffusion of CO_2 from Tissue Cells to Blood

Topic: Part 1 of this Chapter is Simple

The $PaCO_2$ in arterial blood is normally about 40 mmHg. The various feedbacks that control alveolar ventilation (Chapter 11) operate mainly to adjust $PaCO_2$ to this value, so it is normally quite stable at 40 mmHg, even during fairly intense exercise. The PCO_2 in metabolizing tissue cells averages about 46 mmHg when a person is at rest and higher during exercise. Thus, there is a PCO_2 gradient forcing diffusion of CO_2 from tissue cells to blood. CO_2 diffuses very rapidly and by the time blood has passed through the microcirculation PCO_2 is the same in blood plasma and red cells as it is in the tissue cells. Mixed venous blood has a PCO_2 of 46 mmHg in a normal person at rest.

Part 2: Paths Taken by CO_2 after Entering Blood

Topic 1: General

After CO_2 enters blood it follows several paths:

- About 8% remains in plasma:
  o Some of this is hydrated in plasma to carbonic acid which ionizes to bicarbonate and hydrogen ions.
  o A tiny bit combines with terminal amino groups on plasma proteins to form carbamino compounds.
  o The rest remains as dissolved CO_2.

- About 92% diffuses on into red cells where it has three fates:
  o By far the most important is the carbonic anhydrase reaction followed by the chloride shift.
  o Of considerable importance is the carbamino-hemoglobin reaction.
  o Of some importance is dissolved CO_2 in red cell cytoplasm.

Topic 2: Detail   Figure1

CO_2 Dissolved in Plasma (3%)
The solubility coefficient for CO_2 in blood plasma at 37° C is 0.059 ml_{CO2}/dl_{blood}/mmHg. Therefore, at a PCO_2 of 46 mmHg plasma contains 2.7 ml/dl of dissolved CO_2. This can be compared to the dissolved O_2 content in plasma at 100 mmHg, which is only 0.3 ml/dl. Thus, dissolved CO_2 in blood has a more important role than dissolved O_2.

Conversion of CO_2 to bicarbonate in plasma (5%)
CO_2 is spontaneously hydrated in plasma to form HCO_3^- and H^+. The reaction takes place in two steps:

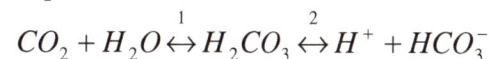

$$CO_2 + H_2O \overset{1}{\leftrightarrow} H_2CO_3 \overset{2}{\leftrightarrow} H^+ + HCO_3^-$$

Step 1 forms carbonic acid (H_2CO_3) and without carbonic anhydrase step 1 is rather slow. Nevertheless, it is fast enough to handle roughly 5% of metabolic CO_2. Step 2 is the dissociation of carbonic acid to protons and bicarbonate. This reaction is instantaneous and requires no enzyme.

The Carbonic Anhydrase Reaction in Red Cells and the Chloride Shift (70%)

Most CO_2 from metabolizing cells diffuses on into red cells and most of this is converted to HCO_3^- and H^+ by carbonic anhydrase (ca). Carbonic anhydrase is abundant in red cells. It is not significantly present in blood plasma. It catalyzes the reversible hydration of CO_2. The reaction is the same as shown above except that the reversible hydration of CO_2 to H_2CO_3 (step 1) is tremendously faster.

In metabolizing tissues, CO_2 drives the reaction to the right and a proton is generated along with a bicarbonate anion. Does proton release by the carbonic anhydrase reaction acidify the red cells? Not much, because extra H^+ is quickly buffered by Hb. Hemoglobin is a very good H^+ buffer at physiological pH.

The Chloride Shift

In red cell membranes there is a transporter called the anion exchanger 1 (AE1), which catalyzes the exchange of Cl^- for HCO_3^- between inside and outside of red cells. AE1 is an obligatory exchanger, meaning that one anion cannot move unless another moves in the opposite direction. Usually this is Cl^- for HCO_3^-. The AE1 exchanger is very fast. Just as quickly as HCO_3^- is generated in red cells it leaves in exchange for plasma Cl^-.

This is called the chloride shift (originally called the Hamburger shift after the investigator who discovered it). AE1 was originally called band 3 protein owing to its location in gel electrophoresis and this term is still often used. The red cell bilayer membrane itself is essentially impermeable to bicarbonate, so exchange for chloride on AE1 is the only way that bicarbonate generated in the red cell can get out into the plasma.

The Carbamino-Hemoglobin Reaction (20%)

In red cells CO_2 binds to terminal amine groups on globin chains. The reaction is

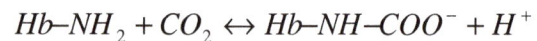

$$Hb–NH_2 + CO_2 \leftrightarrow Hb–NH–COO^- + H^+$$

This reaction occurs rapidly without an enzyme. As CO_2 is generated in metabolizing tissues and then diffuses into red cells, the carbamino-hemoglobin reaction is driven to the right by mass action. Note that a proton is generated when the reaction goes to the right. Again, the generation of H^+ by the carbamino-hemoglobin reaction in red cells changes red cell pH very little because of the large buffering capacity of Hb. The carbamino reaction also occurs with plasma proteins such as albumin but, quantitatively, this is not significant.

Dissolved CO_2 in Red Cells (2%)

This value assumes the same solubility coefficient in red cells as in plasma.

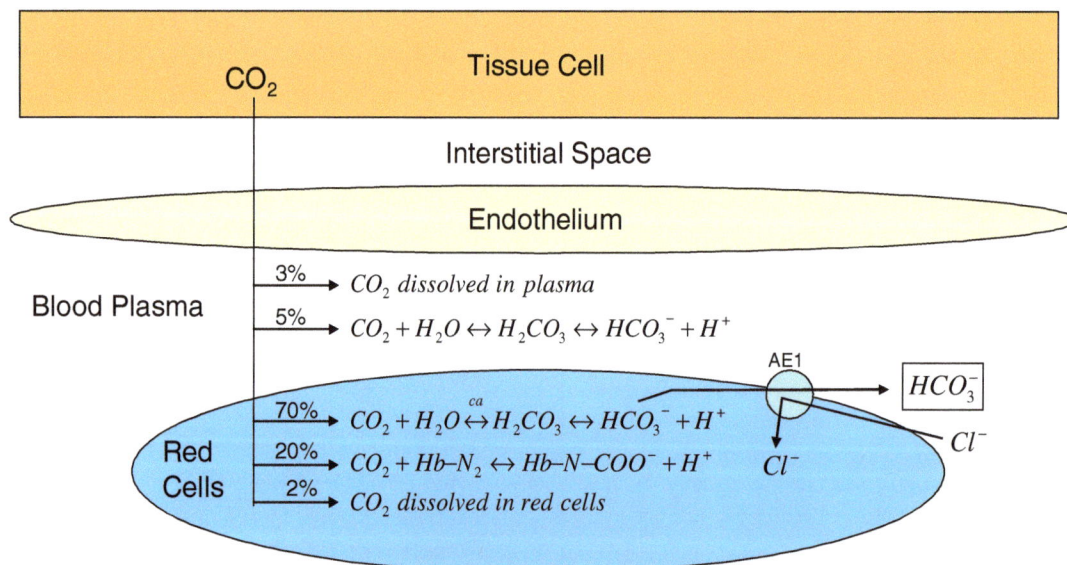

Figure 1. Shown here are the paths taken by CO_2 after being generated by metabolism in tissue cells. The quantitative importance of each path is indicated as a percentage (very approximate). Note that by far the greatest percentage of CO_2 (~70%) is converted to HCO_3^- in red cells by the carbonic anhydrase (ca) reaction and is then transferred back to plasma in exchange for Cl^- (the chloride shift, see text). AE1 is the obligatory Cl^--HCO_3^- exchanger.

Part 3: Paths Taken by CO_2 in the Lungs

Topic 1: Reversal of Peripheral Paths

In the lungs, as CO_2 diffuses into the alveoli and blood PCO_2 declines from 46 to 40 mmHg, all of the above reactions reverse simply because of mass action.

1. Dissolved CO_2 diffuses from plasma to alveoli and from red cells to plasma.
2. Decreased red cell CO_2 causes the carbonic anhydrase reaction to go to the left. This forms more dissolved CO_2 which diffuses out and also reduces the concentration of HCO_3^-
3. Decreased intracellular HCO_3^- causes the chloride shift to operate in reverse with HCO_3^- moving in and Cl^- moving out.
4. The HCO_3^- that has reentered red cells combines with H^+ to form CO_2 by the carbonic anhydrase reaction. This CO_2 diffuses out of the red cells and on into the alveoli.
5. The carbamino reaction reverses, supplying more CO_2 to diffuse into the alveoli.

Topic 2: Why the Chloride Shift?

It seems odd that in the lungs plasma HCO_3^- must move into red cells on AE1 before it can be converted back to CO_2, but this is where the carbonic anhydrase is located. It might seem simpler to put the carbonic anhydrase in plasma. Why not? There are at least two reasons that carbonic anhydrase is more advantageously located in red cells than in plasma: 1) that is where the great H^+ buffering power of hemoglobin is located, and 2) that is where the buffering of H^+ by hemoglobin produces the Bohr effect (increased acidity causes increased release of oxygen from hemoglobin). Another possible reason is that carbonic anhydrase circulating in plasma would have access to all sorts of things that it might harm.

Optional:
But is the chloride shift really necessary? I can't answer this question, but it has been seriously asked in the past. AE1 in red cell membranes is important for helping to hold the cytoskeleton together (see any cell biology text), but is its anion exchange function essential? Why not just carry the bicarbonate back to the lungs within the red cells?

Part 4: The CO_2 Dissociation Curve

Topic 1: Basics

Figure 2
A plot of CO_2 volume carried in 100 ml of blood as a function of PCO_2 is called a CO_2 dissociation curve. Normal CO_2 dissociation curves for arterial blood and for venous blood are shown in Figure 2.

Unlike Hb-O_2 dissociation curves, CO_2 dissociation curves are not sigmoidal and they do not saturate. The important point is that as PCO_2 rises (due to metabolism), more CO_2 can be carried away in blood.

The most interesting thing about these dissociation curves is that the curve for venous blood is higher than that for arterial blood. This has to do entirely with the amount of O_2 bound to Hb. As O_2 leaves Hb in the tissues, blood is able to carry more CO_2 at any given PCO_2. This is called the <u>Haldane effect</u>, which is described in the next topic.

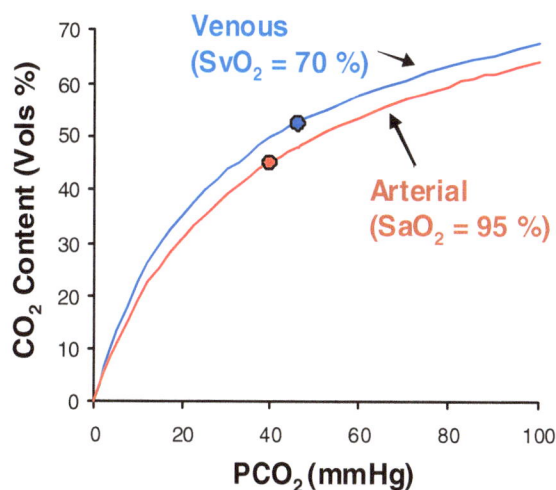

Figure 2. CO_2 dissociation curves for arterial and venous blood. Blue point is operating point in venous blood, red point is operating point in arterial blood.

Optional:

The CO_2 dissociation curve, while it looks simple, is really rather complex. It is the sum of four saturation curves plus the linear relation between dissolved CO_2 and PCO_2. The saturation curves are:

- Hydration of CO_2 in plasma
- The carbamino reaction with plasma proteins (quantitatively insignificant)
- Hydration of CO_2 in red cells (carbonic anhydrase reaction)
- The carbamino reaction with Hb in red cells

The composite curve doesn't saturate because the dissolved CO_2 curve doesn't saturate. Since the composite curve doesn't saturate, there is no point in plotting percent saturation or defining a P_{50}.

The CO_2 hydration curves saturate because H^+ buffering capacity eventually runs out. The carbamino reaction curve saturates because of limited terminal amine sites.

Topic 2: The Haldane Effect

As Hb loses oxygen in the tissues, blood takes on more carbon dioxide at any given PCO_2. This is the Haldane effect. Look at Figure 2. When arterial blood with an oxygen saturation of 95% comes into a tissue, it would take up about 3.0 ml of CO_2/dl if nothing else happened. To see this, ride the red curve in Figure 2 from $PCO_2 = 40$ mmHg (red dot) to $PCO_2 = 46$ mmHg. But 3.0 ml/dl is not enough. Even at rest, CO_2 is being generated faster than this. But we don't have to take the red curve. Instead of riding the red curve, the CO_2 content goes to the blue dot on the blue curve. This provides an additional 4.5 ml/dl of CO_2 carrying capacity, bringing the total to about 7.5 ml/dl. Thus, in this example, the Haldane effect accounts for about 60% of the CO_2 carried away from metabolizing tissues!

Mechanism of the Haldane Effect

Let's look at the two CO_2 reactions in red cells again. They are the carbonic anhydrase reaction and the carbamino-hemoglobin reaction.

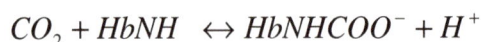

$$CO_2 + H_2O \leftrightarrow HCO_3^- + H^+$$

$$CO_2 + HbNH \leftrightarrow HbNHCOO^- + H^+$$

These reactions both generate hydrogen ions. If H^+ could be gobbled up somehow, both of these reactions would be driven to the right. This is just what happens when O_2 dissociates from hemoglobin; Hb becomes a weaker acid, meaning that it binds hydrogen ions. In the tissues, as O_2 leaves Hb, hydrogen ions bind to hemoglobin and more CO_2 is converted to bicarbonate and to carbaminohemoglobin. This is the Haldane effect.

In the lungs, the reverse happens. O_2 binds to Hb which then becomes a stronger acid, releasing hydrogen ions. This drives the above two reaction to the left; CO_2 is formed and diffuses on into the alveoli. This is also the Haldane effect.

Relation of the Haldane Effect to the Bohr Effect

The Haldane Effect and the Bohr Effect are two sides of the same coin. Both depend on the fact that oxygenated Hb is a stronger acid than is deoxygenated Hb.

Chapter 9

Shunts and $\dot{V}/\dot{Q}$ Mismatching

Part 1: Anatomic Shunts

Part 2: Effect of the $\dot{V}/\dot{Q}$ Ratio on Alveolar Gas Concentrations

Part 3: Effect of the $\dot{V}/\dot{Q}$ Ratio on Oxygen and Carbon Dioxide Delivery to the Systemic Circulation

Part 4: What Can Go Wrong?

Part 1: Anatomic Shunts

Topic 1: Normal Anatomic Shunts

As discussed in Chapter 5, at least half the blood flowing through the bronchial arteries enters the pulmonary veins *via* bronchial-pulmonary anastomoses. This venous blood slightly dilutes the arterialized blood flowing toward the left heart and reduces its O_2 content and PO_2. Arterial PO_2 is affected out of proportion to arterial O_2 content since at the high end of the Hb-O_2 dissociation curve a small change in O_2 content results in a large change in PO_2 (see Chapter 7).

Another normal anatomic shunt is coronary blood that returns to the left ventricle *via* Thebesian veins, again slightly reducing the O_2 content of blood that had been arterialized in the lungs.

Topic 2: Pathological Anatomic Shunts

Pathological Extrapulmonary Shunts

Right-to-left shunts can occur under some circumstances through a patent ductus arteriosus, foramen ovale, ventricular septal defect, or in tetralogy of Fallot.

Pathological Intrapulmonary Shunts

Sometimes there are anastomoses between small pulmonary arteries and veins. Blood taking this path never exchanges O_2 or CO_2 with alveolar air and constitutes a shunt.

In many pulmonary diseases, some alveoli are not ventilated due to bronchiolar blockage or collapse. The air in these alveoli quickly comes into equilibrium with pulmonary arterial blood. The blood flowing around these alveoli, therefore, does not gain any O_2 or lose any CO_2 and is simply shunted to the pulmonary veins without becoming arterialized. Diseases that can lead to this kind of shunt include emphysema, bronchitis, pneumonia, cystic fibrosis, and asthma. The same effect occurs when alveoli are filled with fluid (alveolar edema), and also when they are collapsed (atelectasis).

Atelectasis can be caused by surfactant deficiency as in the respiratory distress syndrome common in premature babies. It can also be caused by pneumothorax; this is called compression atelectasis. Atelectasis frequently occurs after airway blockage. In this case alveolar gas is gradually absorbed into blood over a period of hours to days and it is called absorption atelectasis. The mechanism of absorption atelectasis is complex, but is probably driven by a slow absorption of O_2 down its partial pressure gradient.

Partial Intrapulmonary Shunts

The above situations are all examples of complete shunt (also called absolute shunt or true shunt) in which some blood passes from the right side of the heart to the left without ever having a chance to become even slightly arterialized. But, clearly, if some alveoli are poorly ventilated but are well perfused with blood, the blood flowing around them will be poorly arterialized and behave as though it is partially shunted. Hypoxic vasoconstriction can reduce the effect of partial intrapulmonary shunting by reducing blood flow to poorly ventilated alveoli, but this cannot completely correct the problem.

If a patient has low arterial PO_2 (hypoxemia), a good test for the possibility that complete shunt is the cause is to have the patient breathe 100% O_2. There will be hardly any increase in arterial PO_2 since the shunted blood is not affected by the increase in PO_2 of ventilated alveoli. With partial shunt due to low $\dot{V}/\dot{Q}$ ratio (see below) breathing 100% O_2 does raise arterial PO_2 to some degree.

Topic 3: The Shunt Equation

Total cardiac output (Q_T) is the sum of shunt flow (Q_S) and normal flow (Q_N).

$$Q_T = Q_S + Q_N$$

> [The term "normal flow" should be interpreted to mean flow around normally ventilated alveoli.]

The rates of O_2 delivery to the aorta are given by flow rates multiplied by O_2 concentrations. Therefore,

$$Q_T \cdot CaO_2 = Q_S \cdot CvO_2 + Q_N \cdot C_N O_2$$

> CaO_2 = O_2 concentration in aortic blood
> CvO_2 = O_2 concentration in mixed venous blood
> $C_N O_2$ = O_2 concentration in blood leaving normally ventilated alveoli

Substituting Q_T - Q_S for Q_N and solving for Q_S/Q_T we get

$$\frac{Q_S}{Q_T} = \frac{C_N O_2 - CaO_2}{C_N O_2 - CvO_2}$$

This is the <u>shunt equation</u>. It is correct only if all the shunting is complete. If there is some partial shunting the shunt equation can be interpreted as the hypothetical value of the Q_S/Q_T ratio if all the shunting were complete, and this value can still be useful. How is it useful? It provides a way to assess the extent of the problem.

Note: $C_N O_2$ cannot be directly measured, but it can be estimated from alveolar PO_2 (using the alveolar air equation) and the Hb-O_2 dissociation curve.

[Most readers will probably not be interested in the above derivation, but the shunt equation itself is important.]

Part 2: Effect of the $\dot{V}/\dot{Q}$ Ratio on Alveolar Gas Concentrations

---
Topic 1: Fundamentals

In Chapter 4 we saw that the fractional concentration of CO_2 in alveolar air ($F_A CO_2$) is given by

$$F_A CO_2 = \frac{\dot{V}_E CO_2}{\dot{V}_A}$$

> $\dot{V}_E CO2$ = rate of CO_2 exhaled
>
> $\dot{V}_A$ = rate of alveolar ventilation

This equation will be used here for any single alveolus. We also know that the rate that CO_2 is exhaled from this alveolus is the same as the rate that it enters from alveolar capillary blood, which is

$$\dot{V}_E CO_2 = \dot{Q}\,(CvCO_2 - CaCO_2)$$

> $\dot{Q}$ = Rate of capillary blood flow around this alveolus
> $CvCO_2$ = Concentration of CO_2 in blood entering the capillaries around this alveolus
> $CaCO_2$ = Concentration of CO_2 in arterialized blood leaving this alveolus

Putting these two equations together we get

$$F_A CO_2 = \frac{CvCO_2 - CaCO_2}{\dot{V}/\dot{Q}}$$

Also in Chapter 4 we saw that the fractional concentration of O_2 in alveolar air ($F_A O_2$) is

$$F_A O_2 = FiO_2 - \frac{\dot{V} O_2}{\dot{V}_A}$$

FiO_2 = Fractional concentration of O_2 in humidified inspired air

$\dot{V} O_2$ = Rate of O_2 consumption

The rate of O_2 consumption from this single alveolus is

$$\dot{V} O_2 = \dot{Q} (CaO_2 - CvO_2)$$

Therefore,

$$F_A O_2 = FiO_2 - \frac{CaO_2 - CvO_2}{\dot{V}/\dot{Q}}$$

The above derivation is probably not of much interest to most readers and is given here for the sake of completeness. But, a remarkable conclusion is evident from the two boxed equations above. Read on.

Topic 2: Alveolar PO₂ and PCO₂

Figure 1
These two equations show that the concentrations and, therefore, partial pressures of O_2 and CO_2 in any alveolus depend on the ratio of ventilation to perfusion: the $\dot{V}/\dot{Q}$ ratio. The amazing thing is that it makes no difference whether the ratio is changed by a change in ventilation or a change in perfusion, or both. It is only the ratio that matters. If the $\dot{V}/\dot{Q}$ ratio increases, alveolar PO₂ goes up and PCO₂ goes down as shown in Figure 1.

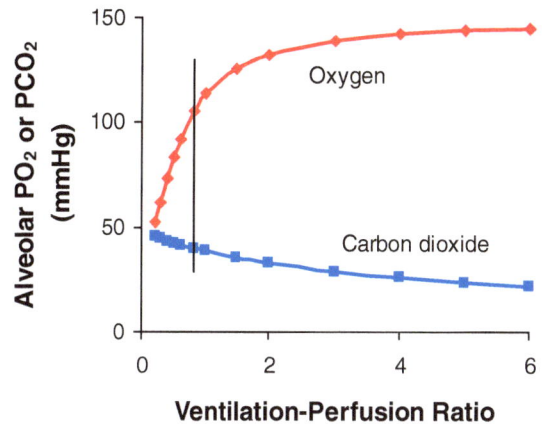

Figure 1. Alveolar PO₂ and PCO₂ as a function of the $\dot{V}/\dot{Q}$ ratio plotted according to the two boxed equations on this page. It is assumed that CvO₂ is constant at 15 vols%, CvCO₂ is constant at 52.6 vols%, FiO₂ is 20%, and atmospheric pressure is 760 mmHg. The vertical line is at normal $\dot{V}/\dot{Q}$ ratio for the entire lungs.

Note the following points:
- If the $\dot{V}/\dot{Q}$ ratio for any alveolus becomes zero, owing to no ventilation because of blockage or collapse, we have a complete shunt since there would be no gas exchange.
- With $\dot{V}/\dot{Q}$ ratios somewhat above zero we can have a partial shunt since blood would get through without being properly arterialized.
- With an infinitely high $\dot{V}/\dot{Q}$ ratio, owing to no blood flow, the affected alveoli become alveolar dead space since they are ventilated but there is no gas exchange. [Remember from Chapter 4 that alveolar dead space plus anatomic dead space is called the physiologic dead space.]
- With very high $\dot{V}/\dot{Q}$ ratios, there could be far too little blood getting through to carry much oxygen and such an alveolus, would be, in effect, partially dead space.

Topic 3: Classic O₂-CO₂ Diagram

Figure 2
There is a traditional way of illustrating the same information shown in Figure 1. It is called the alveolar O₂-CO₂ diagram. A modified version is shown in Figure 2.

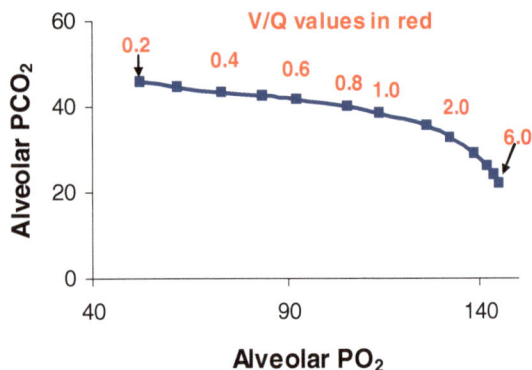

Figure 2. The alveolar O_2-CO_2 diagram.

For any given $\dot{V}/\dot{Q}$ ratio, one can read off the alveolar PO_2 and PCO_2 values. [Frankly, I find this way of presenting the information a little confusing, but students should probably be aware of it.]

Topic 4: The Apex to Base Gradient for the $\dot{V}/\dot{Q}$ Ratio

Recall from Chapter 4 that as the lungs are descended the $\dot{V}/\dot{Q}$ ratio decreases. At the apex (upright person) the $\dot{V}/\dot{Q}$ ratio may be as high as 3.3 and, therefore, alveolar PO_2 will be relatively high and PCO_2 relatively low. At the base the $\dot{V}/\dot{Q}$ ratio is roughly 0.6 and PO_2 is expected to be somewhat low and PCO_2 somewhat high.

Part 3: Effect of the $\dot{V}/\dot{Q}$ Ratio on Oxygen and Carbon Dioxide Delivery to the Systemic Circulation

Topic: O_2 and CO_2 Delivery

Figure 3

We will assume that alveolar capillary blood comes to equilibrium with alveolar O_2 so that when this blood leaves any particular alveolus it has the same PO_2 that is in that alveolus. Next we calculate the content of O_2 in this blood using the Hb-O_2 dissociation curve (Chapter 7). Delivery of O_2 per minute from this alveolus to the pulmonary veins and beyond is given by O_2 concentration multiplied by flow rate. O_2 delivery as a function of the $\dot{V}/\dot{Q}$ ratio is shown in Figure 3. Delivery is expressed as volume per minute relative to that at a $\dot{V}/\dot{Q}$ ratio of 0.8.

For oxygen delivery, it makes a great deal of difference whether the $\dot{V}/\dot{Q}$ ratio is changed by a change in ventilation or a by change in perfusion. Consider the red curve in Figure 3. Here ventilation was changed with perfusion constant. With increasing ventilation there is an increase in O_2 delivery, but this increase is very small at $\dot{V}/\dot{Q}$ ratios greater than 0.8. The blue curve shows that when $\dot{V}/\dot{Q}$ is increased by decreasing perfusion, there is a major decrease in O_2 delivery. These results are probably intuitively obvious, at least qualitatively: more ventilation leads to more O_2

delivery, and less perfusion leads to less O_2 delivery.

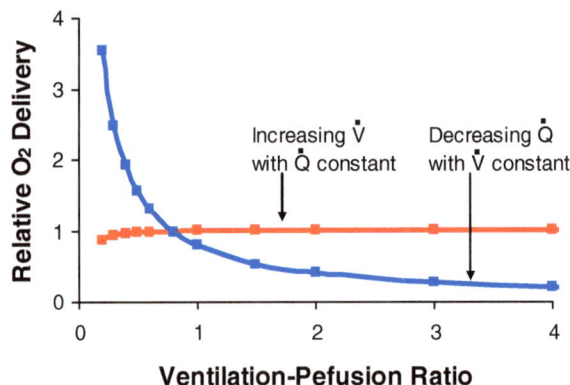

Figure 3. Relative oxygen delivery to pulmonary veins as a function of the $\dot{V}/\dot{Q}$ ratio. The red points show the effect of changing the $\dot{V}/\dot{Q}$ ratio by changing ventilation with perfusion constant. The blue points show the effect of changing the $\dot{V}/\dot{Q}$ ratio by changing perfusion with ventilation constant.

Figure 4

We can do the same thing for CO_2, using the CO_2 dissociation curve (Chapter 8) to get CO_2 content in the blood leaving any particular alveolus. Figure 4 shows CO_2 delivered to the pulmonary veins and beyond as a function of the $\dot{V}/\dot{Q}$ ratio. Delivery is expressed as volume per minute relative to that at a $\dot{V}/\dot{Q}$ ratio of 0.8.

Here again, the results are qualitatively intuitive: more ventilation leads to less CO_2 delivery to the pulmonary veins and less perfusion also leads to less CO_2 delivery.

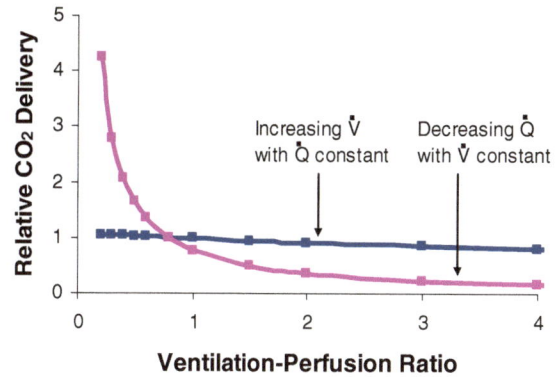

Figure 4. Carbon dioxide delivery as a function of the $\dot{V}/\dot{Q}$ ratio.

Part 4: What Could Possibly Go Wrong?

Pathological Extrapulmonary Shunts
- Patent ductus arteriosus
- Patent foramen ovale
- Ventricular septal defect.

Pathological Intrapulmonary Shunts
- Arterio-Venous Anastomoses
- Complete Bronchial or Bronchiolar Blockage or Collapse
  - Foreign object
  - Tumor
  - Emphysema
  - Chronic bronchitis
  - Pneumonia
  - Cystic fibrosis
  - Asthma
- Alveolar Blockage or Collapse
  - Pulmonary edema (see Chapter 4)
  - Atelectasis
    - Surfactant deficiency
    - Compression atelectasis
    - Absorption atelectasis

Abnormal Degrees of $\dot{V}/\dot{Q}$ Mismatch
- Reduced Ventilation (low $\dot{V}/\dot{Q}$)
  - COPD (because of blockage and collapse of airways – some more than others)
  - ARDS (due to collapse of alveoli and pulmonary edema)
  - IRDS (due to collapse of alveoli and pulmonary edema)
  - Fibrotic lung disease (due to regional variations in compliance)

- Reduced Perfusion (high $\dot{V}/\dot{Q}$)
  - Pulmonary emboli
  - Circulatory shock
  - Eisenmenger's syndrome (increased pulmonary vascular resistance)

Arterial Hypoxemia
  - Decreased FiO_2
  - Hypoventilation
  - Diffusion impairment
  - Abnormal shunts
  - Abnormal degrees of V/Q mismatch

A more complete list of the causes of arterial hypoxemia is given in Chapter 9.

Chapter 10

The Causes of Arterial Hypoxemia and Hypercapnia

Part 1: Hypoxemia
Part 2: Hypercapnia
Part 3: What Can Go Wrong?

Part 1: Hypoxemia

Topic 1: Introduction

Abnormally low arterial PO_2 is often not apparent, except by blood gas analysis, until it gets below roughly 60 mmHg. At this value hemoglobin is still about 90% saturated. Severe arterial hypoxemia (*e.g.* < 40 mmHg) can result in malfunction of many organs because of tissue hypoxia. The central nervous system and the heart are especially vulnerable. Cyanosis and lactic acidosis are important signs of severe arterial hypoxemia.

The difference between PO_2 in alveoli and arterial blood, the A-a PO_2 difference, is a very important measurement. Arterial PO_2 is determined by routine blood gas analysis. The alveolar air equation (Chapter 4) is used to determine alveolar PO_2. Normally, arterial PO_2 is a few mmHg less than alveolar PO_2. This difference is caused by normal anatomic shunts and a normal degree of $\dot{V}/\dot{Q}$ mismatch. It increases with age. A rule of thumb for aging is that the A-a PO_2 difference should not be greater than about age/4 + 4 mmHg. A slightly different rule of thumb is that PaO_2 should be at least 100 – age/3 mmHg.

Note: A-a PO_2 <u>difference</u> is the correct terminology. However, the term <u>gradient</u> is often used in this connection even though a gradient is defined as a difference in some property between two locations divided by the distance between them, *i.e.* a slope.

Topic 2: The Causes of Arterial Hypoxemia

There are five general causes of arterial hypoxemia. The final three can also lead to an abnormal increase in the A-a PO_2 difference.

1. <u>Low FiO_2</u> as in mountain climbing or flying at altitude without a pressurized cabin.
2. <u>Low alveolar ventilation</u> (hypoventilation)

- Restrictive pulmonary diseases
- Obstructive pulmonary diseases
- Pneumothorax
- Drugs that cause respiratory depression (*e.g.* narcotics)

A somewhat more detailed list of the causes of hypoventilation is given in Chapter 4.

3. <u>Diffusion impairment</u>
- Interstitial fibrosis
- Scleroderma
- Pulmonary edema

Diffusion impairment is rarely an important cause of arterial hypoxemia except to some extent during exercise in patients having diffusion impairment, and in extremely advanced cases of interstitial fibrosis.

4. <u>Abnormal shunts</u>
- Congenital heart defects
- Blockage of bronchi by foreign objects

5. <u>Abnormal degrees of $\dot{V}/\dot{Q}$ mismatch</u>
- COPD (emphysema and chronic bronchitis)
- ARDS (adult respiratory distress syndrome, also called acute respiratory distress syndrome)
- IRDS (infant respiratory distress syndrome)
- Asthma
- Pulmonary embolism
- Oxygen toxicity (which may cause atelectasis).

Of these causes of arterial hypoxemia, hypoventilation and abnormal $\dot{V}/\dot{Q}$ mismatch are by far the most important clinically.

Topic 3: How Does $\dot{V}/\dot{Q}$ Mismatch Cause Arterial Hypoxemia?

The Perfect Lung

First we shall consider the so-called "perfect lung", in which there is no anatomic shunt and all alveoli have the same $\dot{V}/\dot{Q}$ ratio. Let's say that total alveolar ventilation is 4,000 ml/min and total perfusion is 5,000 ml/min resulting in a normal $\dot{V}/\dot{Q}$ ratio of 0.8. Alveolar PO_2 everywhere will be 105 mmHg (according to Figure 1 in Chapter 9). The blood leaving any region of this "perfect lung" will also have a PO_2 of 105 mmHg. Using the Hb-O_2 dissociation curve (Chapter 6) and assuming a hemoglobin concentration of 15.0 mg%, an arterial PO_2 of 105 mmHg translates to an O_2 content of 20 vols%. Since all regions behave identically, the mixed blood in the left heart will also have an O_2 content of 20 vols% and a PO_2 of 105 mmHg.

The Real Lung

In the real lung (still assuming no anatomic shunt) not all alveoli have the same $\dot{V}/\dot{Q}$ ratio. Therefore, blood leaving these alveoli will have various O_2 contents and the O_2 content in the left heart will be an average.

Now let us consider how changes in $\dot{V}/\dot{Q}$ ratios due to changes in 1) regional ventilation and 2) regional perfusion can result in arterial hypoxemia.

Change in $\dot{V}/\dot{Q}$ Ratio Due to Change in Ventilation

There is no problem understanding how a low $\dot{V}/\dot{Q}$ ratio leads to hypoxemia when the low $\dot{V}/\dot{Q}$ ratio is caused by reduced ventilation. With reduced ventilation, PO_2 in the affected alveoli is reduced and, therefore, O_2 delivered per minute or per unit volume of blood is reduced. Of course this tends to lower arterial PO_2.

A high $\dot{V}/\dot{Q}$ ratio due to high ventilation does not in itself lead to hypoxemia. It leads to an increase in alveolar PO_2 and, therefore, in arterial blood PO_2. There is a small increase in O_2 delivery per minute (see Figure 3); this is mainly due to a slight increase in O_2 saturation of hemoglobin with a minor contribution from an increase in dissolved O_2. The increase in O_2 delivery is small even when the rise in PaO_2 is substantial because the Hb-O_2

dissociation curve is nearly flat at its high end. In other words, in this range, a fairly large change in PO_2 causes only a small change in O_2 content.

But what if low ventilation in some alveoli is compensated by high ventilation in other alveoli so that total ventilation is normal? Do the latter make up for the former with regard to arterial PO_2? The answer is no. We will do a calculation similar to the one above for the "perfect lung".

Imagine a hypothetical situation: the lungs have two regions each having the same number of alveoli. Total alveolar ventilation is 4,000 ml/min and total perfusion is 5,000 ml/min giving an overall $\dot{V}/\dot{Q}$ ratio of 0.8. Each region has a blood flow of 2,500 ml/min. Region 1 is hypoventilated at 500 ml/min and has a $\dot{V}/\dot{Q}$ ratio of 0.20. Alveolar PO_2 in region 1 is about 52 mmHg (Figure 1). Therefore, blood leaving region 1 will have an O_2 content of only about 17.6 vols% (from O_2 dissociation curve) instead of the normal 20 vols%. Region 2 is hyperventilated at 3,500 ml/min and has a $\dot{V}/\dot{Q}$ ratio of 1.4. Blood leaving region 2 will have a PO_2 of about 124 mmHg and an O_2 content of about 20.1 vols%. The average $\dot{V}/\dot{Q}$ ratio is normal at 0.8. When the two streams mix we get 17.6 + 20.1 = 37.7 ml of oxygen per 100 ml of blood, or 18.8 vols%. This results in about 94% saturation of hemoglobin and is equivalent to a PO_2 of only about 70 mmHg.

What has happened? Answer: the Hb-O_2 dissociation curve is practically flat at high saturation values, so increasing PO_2 has little effect on O_2 content. At lower saturation values decreasing PO_2 has a much greater effect on O_2 content. So when the streams mix the half coming from low $\dot{V}/\dot{Q}$ alveoli dominates the half coming from high $\dot{V}/\dot{Q}$ alveoli and the resulting O_2 content and, therefore, PO_2 are below normal. The bottom line is that a high $\dot{V}/\dot{Q}$ ratio in half the alveoli cannot compensate for a low $\dot{V}/\dot{Q}$ ratio in the other half.

The general conclusion is that the more variation in the $\dot{V}/\dot{Q}$ ratio above and below the average, the more is the reduction in arterial PO_2!

Change in $\dot{V}/\dot{Q}$ Ratio Due to Change in Perfusion

<u>High</u> $\dot{V}/\dot{Q}$ ratio because of low perfusion leads to hypoxemia. This one is easy. Consider the extreme. If some region of lung has no blood flow, no O_2 will be delivered from this region. These alveoli will contribute to physiologic dead space. At lesser degrees of perfusion impairment, some O_2 will be delivered (see Figure 3) but not a normal amount.

<u>Low</u> $\dot{V}/\dot{Q}$ ratio because of high perfusion also leads to hypoxemia. This is a little difficult to understand since, as shown in Figure 3, O_2 delivery per minute increases steeply as the $\dot{V}/\dot{Q}$ ratio decreases below 0.8. How is increased O_2 delivery/min consistent with decreased arterial PO_2? The answer lies in the fact that increased perfusion, while delivering more O_2 per minute, delivers it at a lower PO_2. This is because at a low $\dot{V}/\dot{Q}$ ratio, alveolar PO_2 goes down (Figure 1).

Again imagine that the lungs are divided into two regions, each the same size and both having the same rate of ventilation, 2,000 ml/min. Region 1 has a perfusion of 4,000 ml/min giving a $\dot{V}/\dot{Q}$ ratio of 0.5. Region 2 has a perfusion of 1,000 ml/min giving a $\dot{V}/\dot{Q}$ ratio of 2.0. According to Figure 1, region 1 has an alveolar PO_2 of about 83.4 mmHg and, therefore, delivers blood having a PO_2 of 83.4 mmHg. Region 2 delivers blood at a PO_2 of 132.3 mmHg. Using the Hb-O_2 dissociation curve these PO_2 values translate to 19.26 and 19.79 vols%

respectively. Thus, total O_2 delivery in the mixed blood from these two sources is 19.26 x 40 + 19.79 x 10 = 948.3 ml of O_2 in 5,000 ml of blood. The O_2 concentration in this blood is, therefore, 18.97 vols%. This is about 94.8% saturation and translates to a PO_2 of about 74 mmHg.

We could go through more calculations at various degrees of $\dot{V}/\dot{Q}$ mismatch and at various average $\dot{V}/\dot{Q}s$, but why bother? The general conclusion is clear: the more variation in the $\dot{V}/\dot{Q}$ ratio above and below the mean, the more the reduction in arterial PO_2!

Low Alveolar Ventilation Combined with $\dot{V}/\dot{Q}$ Mismatch

Many pulmonary diseases result in reduced alveolar ventilation in addition to $\dot{V}/\dot{Q}$ mismatch. Consider lungs with a total alveolar ventilation of only 2,000 ml/min but a total perfusion of 5,000 ml/min resulting in an overall $\dot{V}/\dot{Q}$ ratio of 0.4. If both ventilation and perfusion are uniformly distributed we can calculate that arterial PO_2 will be 73 mmHg. However, if the distribution of ventilation is uniform but the distribution of perfusion is 4 to 1, we can calculate that arterial PO_2 will be only about 62 mmHg.

Part 2: Hypercapnia

Topic 1: Hypoventilation

The main cause of hypercapnia is hypoventilation. In fact hypoventilation is defined as a rate of alveolar ventilation less than that necessary to meet metabolic needs, signified by a $PaCO_2$ > 45 mmHg. Hypoventilation can occur in a variety of disorders including polio, amyotrophic lateral sclerosis, myasthenia gravis, chronic bronchitis, emphysema, asthma, *etc*.

Topic 2: How Does $\dot{V}/\dot{Q}$ Mismatch Affect Arterial PCO_2?

We can go through the same line of reasoning and calculations that we did for oxygen, with regions 1 and 2 having $\dot{V}/\dot{Q}$ ratios of 0.2 and 1.4 respectively due to a difference in alveolar ventilation with uniform perfusion. Alveolar PCO_2 will be about 46 and 36 mmHg respectively. According to the CO_2 dissociation curve in Chapter 7, the CO_2 contents in blood leaving regions 1 and 2 will be about 52 and 46 vols% respectively.

When the two streams mix, the result will be 49 vols%, which translates to a PCO_2 of about 41 mmHg. This is only slightly above the normal value of 40 mmHg. The reason that the effect is very small is due to the steepness and relative linearity of the CO_2 dissociation curve – a given change in CO_2 content does not produce as large a change in partial pressure as does the same change in O_2 content.

In addition, the main signal that normally controls alveolar ventilation is arterial PCO_2 (see Chapter 11). Any elevation in arterial PCO_2 results in a reflex increase in alveolar ventilation that blows off more CO_2 and gets arterial PCO_2 back to normal. Thus, $\dot{V}/\dot{Q}$ mismatches can lead to serious hypoxemia but seldom lead to serious hypercapnia. An exception is in advanced COPD in which significant hypoventilation combines with $\dot{V}/\dot{Q}$ mismatch. In this case, severe hypercapnia with respiratory acidosis can result.

Part 3: What Can Go Wrong?

$\dot{V}/\dot{Q}$ Mismatch
Discussed above and in Chapter 9.

Hypoventilation
Discussed above.

Hyperventilation
Hyperventilation can be voluntary or can occur during anxiety. By definition, hyperventilation results in significantly reduced arterial PCO_2 (hypocapnia). The person can get woozy and even faint. Cerebral blood flow is strongly influenced by PCO_2. Hypercapnia causes increased cerebral blood flow and hypocapnia does the opposite. Thus, hyperventilation reduces cerebral blood flow with consequent reduction in O_2 supply to the brain. It is cerebral hypoxia that causes the symptoms.

Chapter 11

Control of Ventilation

Part 1: Central Control of Rhythmicity

Topic 1: Introduction

Breathing is spontaneous. We don't have to think about it, it just happens in a reasonably regular rhythm, even while we are asleep. We can voluntarily override the natural rhythm for a short time as in talking, singing, and breath holding, but before long it involuntarily kicks in again. The rhythmic automaticity of breathing is rather different from that of the heart beat. In the heart, automaticity is the function of modified cardiac muscle cells, normally the pacemaking cells in the sinoatrial node. On the other hand, rhythmic breathing is controlled by neurons in the brainstem, most importantly in medullary regions collectively called the medullary respiratory center. Frequency and depth of breathing are altered to meet demand by signals sent to the medullary respiratory center from other regions in the medulla that sense acidity directly and arterial PCO_2 indirectly, and also from certain peripheral receptors that detect arterial PO_2, PCO_2, and acidity.

Topic 2: The Centers

Figure 1
It needs to be acknowledged up front that our understanding of central control is sketchy. The locations of the brain stem centers responsible for automatic rhythmic breathing are shown in Figure 1.

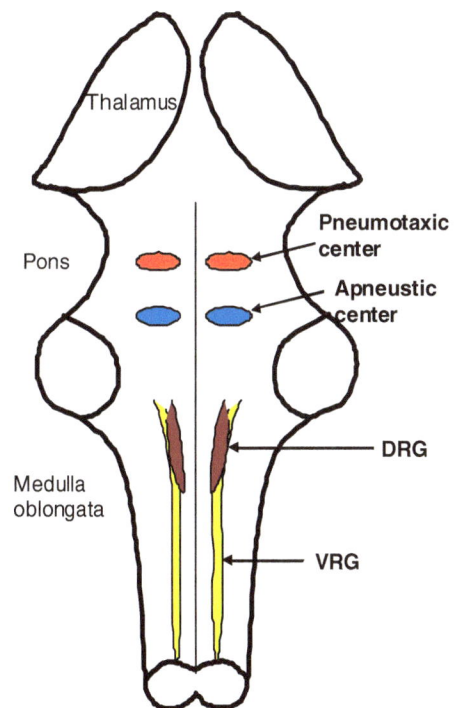

Figure 1. Outline of the brain stem looking from the dorsal side. The approximate locations of the respiratory control groups are indicated.

The Dorsal Respiratory Group

There are bilateral regions in the medulla oblongata called the dorsal respiratory group (DRG). The DRG lies in the reticular formation just below the floor of the 4th ventricle within and around the nucleus of the tractus solitarius (NTS). The NTS is the region that receives afferent input from the lungs, cardiovascular system, and gastrointestinal tract *via* the vagus and glossopharyngeal nerves. The DRG interprets this information and drives inspiration by causing excitation of motor neurons to the diaphragm and to the other muscles of inspiration. The DRG was formerly known as the "inspiratory center"; however, some inspiratory drive is also mediated *via* the ventral respiratory group.

The Ventral Respiratory Group

The ventral respiratory group (VRG) was formerly called the "expiratory center", but it is now known to serve both inspiration and expiration. The VRG is located in and around a long column of anatomically identifiable structures that include the Botzinger complex, the nucleus ambiguous, and the nucleus retroambiguous. The VRG presumably drives active expiration when it is required as in exercise, obstructive pulmonary diseases, coughing, sneezing, playing wind instruments, *etc.*

Rhythmicity

Roughly every five seconds inspiratory muscles are excited with gradually increasing intensity (this is often called a ramp of excitation). After about two seconds excitation rapidly subsides and passive expiration takes place over the next three seconds. We do not understand the mechanism of breathing rhythmicity. It could result from reverberating circuits in the central control regions of the medulla much like reentry pathways in the heart that are responsible for some kinds of arrhythmias. On the other hand, it could result from pacemaking activity in specific groups of neurons much like the situation with nodal pacemaking cells in the heart. Currently, the latter mechanism is widely embraced and the most likely site for pacemaking activity appears to be a region at the rostral end of the VRG called the pre-Botzinger complex.

There are two ways that frequency and depth of breathing can be controlled: 1) changing the slope of the excitatory ramp and 2) changing the duration of the excitatory ramp. For example, if the ramp is terminated early, tidal volume will decrease and frequency will increase. If the ramp is prolonged tidal volume will increase and frequency will decrease. On the other hand, if the ramp becomes steeper, tidal volume increases and if it flattens tidal volume decreases. Such changes in the inspiratory ramp are directed largely by sensory input to the DRG.

Pontine Respiratory Groups

On their own, the medullary respiratory regions result in a roughly regular breathing pattern, but they need some fine tuning. This seems to be the job of two regions in the pons, the apneustic center and the pneumotaxic center. The apneustic center is a poorly defined region in the lower pons that seems to try to lengthen the excitatory ramp generated by medullary neurons. The pneumotaxic center is in the upper pons; it tends to modify the effect of the apneustic center and shortens the ramp. When all of these regions are intact, breathing is spontaneous and regular.

[When the effect of the pneumotaxic center is experimentally removed in animals by transecting midway through the pons, inspiration is prolonged. When the apneustic center is also removed by transecting between the pons and medulla, and also the vagus nerves are cut, inspiration is greatly prolonged until finally an expiratory gasp takes place. This is a breathing pattern called apneustic breathing.]

Input From Higher Centers

Information is relayed from the cerebral cortex (voluntary override), the hypothalamus (emotional responses and body temperature changes), and the limbic system (emotional responses) to the medullary control groups and possibly to the pontine groups.

The cerebral cortex can also send impulses directly to the muscles of respiration, bypassing the brain stem centers, for voluntary control of breathing.

Part 2: Control of Ventilation by Central Chemoreceptors

Topic 1: General

Figure 2

There are bilateral columns of neurons very near the ventrolateral surface of the medulla in a region called the central chemoreceptor area (or chemosensitive area). It is located approximately as shown in Figure 2.

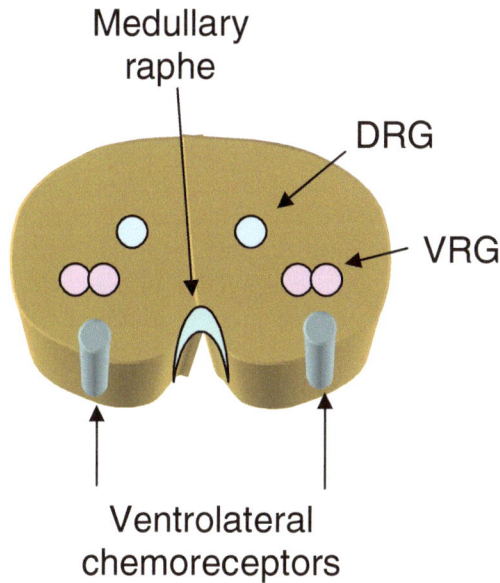

Figure 2. Diagram of cross-section through mid medulla showing location of the ventrolateral chemoreceptors and the medullary raphe. The approximate locations of the DRG and VRG are also indicated for comparison.

Neurons in the central chemoreceptor area sense changes in extracellular acidity and relay this information to the DRG and VRG. Increased acidity (decreased pH) in the interstitial spaces around the neurons of the ventrolateral chemoreceptive area results in increased alveolar ventilation, mainly by increasing tidal volume, but breathing frequency is also increased. Decreased interstitial acidity (increased pH) has the opposite effect. This ventrolateral chemoreceptor area is located very close to the cerebral spinal fluid (CSF) covering the ventral surface of the medulla and it is pH in the CSF that mainly determines interstitial pH in this region.

The pH of the CSF is determined mainly by blood PCO_2. If blood PCO_2 rises, CSF PCO_2 also rises since the blood-CSF barrier is highly permeable to CO_2. As CSF PCO_2 rises its acidity rises because of the familiar CO_2 hydration reaction:

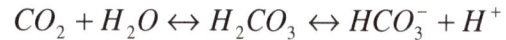

$$CO_2 + H_2O \leftrightarrow H_2CO_3 \leftrightarrow HCO_3^- + H^+$$

So even though the ventrolateral chemoreceptors are directly controlled by pH in the CSF, they are indirectly controlled by blood PCO_2. This is in fact, except during exercise, <u>by far the most important way that alveolar ventilation is normally regulated</u>. If arterial PCO_2 increases, alveolar ventilation increases. This blows off CO_2 until arterial PCO_2 is normal again – obviously a negative feedback cycle. The central chemoreceptors are not very sensitive to blood H^+, since protons cannot readily pass the blood-brain barrier or the blood-CSF barrier.

It is now known that the ventrolateral columns of H^+-sensitive cells are not the only central chemoreceptor regions. There are also groups of highly H^+-sensitive neurons located in other medullary areas, and these also influence pulmonary ventilation. Prominent among these areas are the central medullary raphe, the nucleus ambiguous, and the nucleus tractus solitarius (NTS). There are also cell groups that are thought to be involved in central PCO_2 (acidity) detection in the locus caeruleus, the hypothalamus, and even in the cerebellum. The deeper chemoreceptors are probably influenced directly by blood PCO_2 rather than by CSF PCO_2.

The central chemoreceptors are not appreciably influenced by arterial PO_2, only PCO_2. They may be slightly turned on by low blood pH without elevated $PaCO_2$ as in metabolic acidosis (such as lactic acidosis), but this effect is probably not important. It is the peripheral chemoreceptors (discussed below) that are important for sensing arterial PO_2 and pH. [However if PaO_2 gets really low, the medullary control centers (DRG and VRG) can become greatly depressed, and alveolar ventilation can get critically low.]

The mechanism by which central chemoreceptor neurons detect changes in interstitial pH is not well understood. Reduced pH probably results in depolarization of the receptor neuron cell membrane by inhibiting some type of K^+ channel, but details are not known.

Topic 2: Stimulus-Response Relationship

Figure 3

Figure 3 shows total pulmonary ventilation ($\dot{V}_E$) as a function of arterial PCO_2 (altered by acutely changing PCO_2 in inspired air). Increased $FiCO_2$ causes hypercapnia and consequent respiratory acidosis.

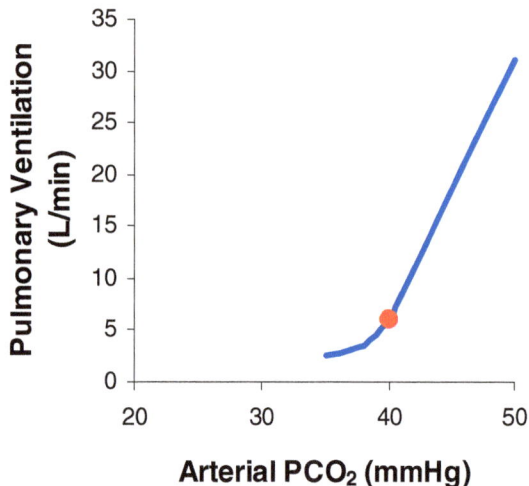

Figure 3. The effect of changing arterial PCO_2 on total pulmonary ventilation. In this experiment $PaCO_2$ was changed by changing the concentration of CO_2 in inspired air ($FiCO_2$). The red dot represents the normal operating point. The rise in $PaCO_2$ above normal reflects a respiratory acidosis. Arterial PO_2 was constant at 100 mmHg.

Pulmonary ventilation increases linearly at $PaCO_2$ values above normal (40 mmHg). This response is rapid in onset but takes a few minutes to become fully developed. It becomes less steep during sleep, with advancing age, and under the influence of CNS depressant drugs such as general anesthetics, ethanol, opiates, and barbiturates.

The ventilatory response to $PaCO_2$ shown in Figure 3 is mostly due to the central chemoreceptors (about 80-90%). The peripheral chemoreceptors (discussed below) account for the rest. They are sensitive to arterial PO_2 and to pH. They also respond to arterial PCO_2, but are relatively unimportant in this respect compared to the central chemoreceptors.

Topic 3: Chronic Hypercapnia and Central Chemoreceptor Adaptation

If hypercapnia continues for more than a day or so, a curious thing happens. The choroid plexus in the cerebral ventricles, which is the main source for secretion of CSF, starts secreting more bicarbonate into the CSF. Bicarbonate is secreted by the choroid plexus by a Na^+-dependent cotransport process. Bicarbonate can actually be secreted uphill against its electrochemical potential gradient. Elevated bicarbonate in the CSF drives the CO_2 hydration reaction to the left, thereby elevating CSF pH back up toward normal. It does not completely reach normal, but the ventilatory drive from arterial PCO_2 on the central chemoreceptors is substantially reduced. The cerebral capillary endothelium (which is the blood-brain barrier) probably also secretes extra bicarbonate into the medullary interstitial spaces, thereby blunting the response of more interior chemoreceptors to arterial CO_2. This happens in patients with chronic hypercapnia due, for example, to emphysema. Consequently, arterial hypoxemia in these patients becomes worse than it would be without this adaptation. With the reduced response of the central chemoreceptors to $PaCO_2$, the respiratory drive in patients with chronic hypercapnia may be mainly a hypoxemic drive from the peripheral chemoreceptors. A dreadful effect can happen if such a patient is suddenly given oxygen to breathe at too high a concentration. This can eliminate the ventilatory drive from the peripheral chemoreceptors. Now without much CO_2 drive from the central chemoreceptors, the patient may become severely apneic, comatose, and possibly die unless the FiO_2 is quickly reduced.

Part 3: Control of Ventilation by Peripheral Chemoreceptors

Topic 1: Peripheral Chemoreceptors

Figure 4

The major peripheral chemoreceptors involved in breathing are the two carotid bodies, each located in the wall of a carotid sinus close to the carotid baroreceptors. There is also a series of aortic chemoreceptors along the inner curvature of the aortic arch. These locations are diagrammed in Figure 4. The carotid bodies send information regarding arterial PO_2, PCO_2 and pH to the central control regions in the medulla. This information is sent *via* the carotid sinus nerve and then on to the glossopharyngeal nerve and the NTS. The aortic bodies send the same sort of information to the central centers *via* the vagus nerve and NTS.

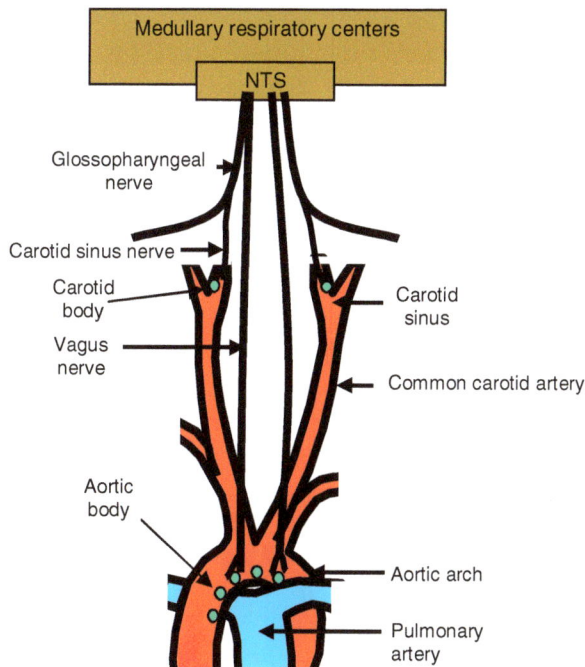

Figure 4. Diagram showing the location of the carotid and aortic bodies and their afferent connections with the NTS.

The aortic bodies are probably not very important regulators of breathing as long as the carotid bodies are functioning properly, but if anything impairs or destroys the carotid bodies, the aortic bodies can up-regulate and take over peripheral breathing control. The rest of this discussion will pertain mainly to the carotid bodies.

Topic 2: Structure and Function of the Carotid Bodies

Figure 5

Figure 5 is a drawing of a section through a carotid body from an old edition of Gray's Anatomy. Diameter is roughly one millimeter. The main receptor cell is called a glomus cell. It is also called a Type I cell. Glomus cells are surrounded by sustentacular cells (Type II cells) which are supporting cells analogous to CNS glial cells.

The carotid bodies are extremely rich with blood vessels. In fact, for their weight, they have the highest blood flow of any organ in the body. Blood flow is so fast through the carotid bodies that hardly any oxygen is used up and the venous blood leaving the carotid bodies has practically arterial composition. So, all the glomus cells detect the same PO_2, PCO_2, and pH.

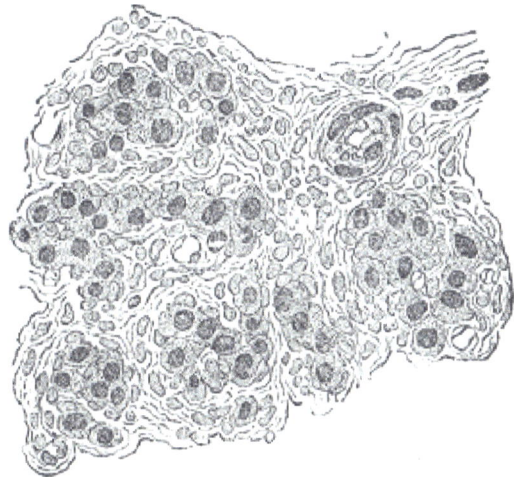

Figure 5. Carotid body from the 1918 edition of Gray's Anatomy.

Figure 6

This is a diagram of the most important elements of arterial PO_2, PCO_2, and pH sensing by the carotid bodies. The glomus cells are the receptors, and they contain a large array of neurotransmitters.

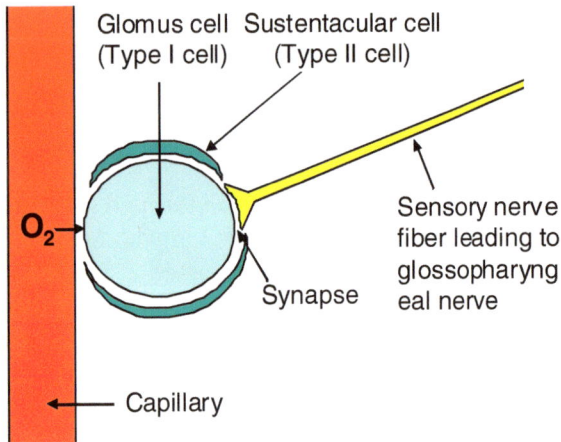

Figure 6. Diagram of the elements involved in sensing arterial PO_2, PCO_2, and pH by the carotid bodies. The glomus cells are also innervated by preganglionic sympathetic nerve fibers (not shown in the figure) which perhaps regulate sensitivity to O_2, CO_2, and pH.

Topic 3: Mechanism of Signal Transduction

Decreased arterial PO_2, increased arterial PCO_2, and decreased arterial pH all result in depolarization of the glomus cell membrane, probably by inhibiting some K^+ channel. Details are not understood. The resulting depolarization leads to Ca^{++} influx which, in turn, triggers release of various neurotransmitters into the synaptic cleft. One or more of these transmitters excites the sensory nerve ending and a signal is transmitted to the medullary DRG. The most important transmitter is probably dopamine.

Topic 4: Stimulus-Response Relationships

The firing frequency of the sinus nerves leaving the carotid bodies increases as arterial PO_2 decreases, PCO_2 increases, or pH decreases. In all three cases the effect on breathing is to increase minute volume by increasing both tidal volume and breathing frequency. Of these three stimuli, PO_2 is the most important since the central chemoreceptors can respond adequately to increases in PCO_2 without much help from peripheral chemoreceptors.

Figure 7

This figure shows the firing frequency in the carotid sinus nerve as arterial PO_2 is changed.

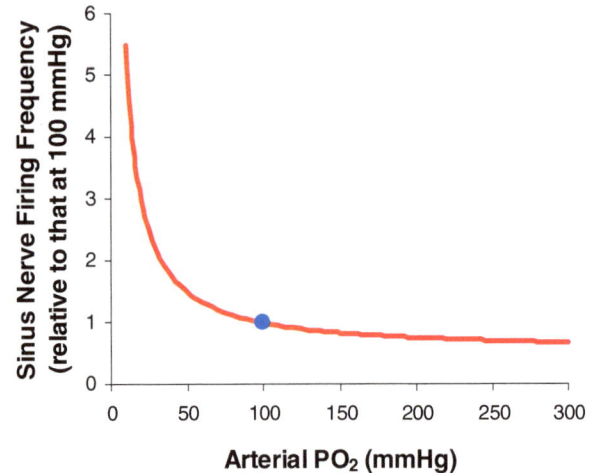

Figure 7. Effect of arterial PO_2 on sinus nerve firing frequency. The frequency data are relative to that at a PO_2 of 100 mmHg which is assigned a value of 1.0 (blue dot).

Note that there is only a small increase in firing frequency as PaO_2 declines until it drops roughly below 60 mmHg. In other words, the carotid bodies are not very sensitive to high PaO_2 or even to mild hypoxemia; but when hypoxemia gets severe, the carotid bodies send a strong positive signal to the medullary centers. It is very interesting that 60 mmHg is approximately the region on the O_2-Hb dissociation curve (Chapter 6) below which hemoglobin gives up large amounts of O_2. The result is that as long as hemoglobin is still carrying plenty of O_2 breathing is not stimulated much, but when PO_2 falls enough to desaturate hemoglobin to a dangerous degree, breathing is stimulated in an attempt to raise PaO_2 back up to an acceptable level.

It is worth noting, however, that even though impulse frequency is not very sensitive to increases in PaO_2 above normal, there is always some input from the carotid bodies to the medullary center even at very high PaO_2 values. It is thought, therefore, that the carotid bodies provide a continuous drive to breathe.

The peripheral chemoreceptors also respond to abnormally high $PaCO_2$ (hypercapnia) and to low arterial H^+ concentration (acidosis). These responses are fairly linear and not nearly as steep as the response to severe hypoxemia. The response to hypercapnia is of dubious importance as long as the central chemoreceptors are functioning properly. The response to acidosis may be important when it is a metabolic acidosis since in this case the increase in H⁺ concentration is not accompanied by hypercapnia as it is in respiratory acidosis. Instead, $PaCO_2$ is usually less than normal in metabolic acidosis because of compensation by

hyperventilation. We will discuss acid-base balance more thoroughly in Chapter 12.

Part 4: Integrated Responses

Topic 1: Combined Changes in PaO_2 and $PaCO_2$

Figure 8
Ordinarily, of course, both the central and peripheral chemoreceptors operate at the same time and now we must examine their combined contributions to pulmonary ventilation. Figure 8 shows how changing PaO_2 influences pulmonary ventilation at two different levels of $PaCO_2$.

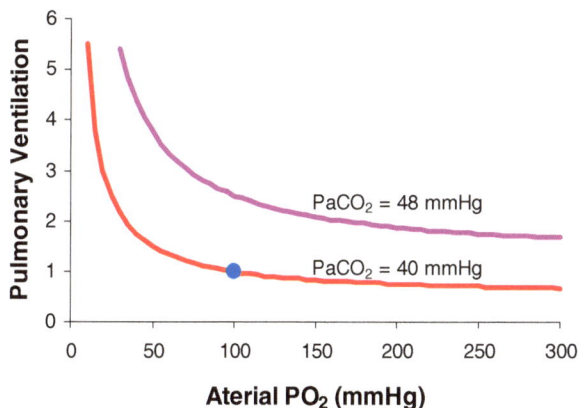

Figure 8. Pulmonary ventilation as a function of PaO_2 at two different levels of $PaCO_2$. The pulmonary ventilation values are relative to that at $PaO_2 = 100$ mmHg and $PaCO_2 = 40$ mmHg.

Note that at any value for PaO_2, ventilation is increased when $PaCO_2$ is increased. This effect is mainly due to the effect of $PaCO_2$ on the central chemoreceptors but is helped somewhat by the peripheral chemoreceptors.

Topic 2: Metabolic Acidosis

This topic is important in the present context but will not be discussed until Chapter 12.

Topic 3: Exercise

The hyperpnea of exercise, after at least a century of investigation, is still a mystery; a mystery that

has vexed many highly accomplished physiologists over the years.

Up to roughly 50-70% of maximum O_2 consumption, alveolar ventilation increases in proportion to the increased rates of oxygen consumption and carbon dioxide production. What drives this increase in ventilation? In all but the most intense and prolonged exercise, $PaCO_2$ does not increase nor does PaO_2 decrease. With very intense and prolonged exercise, $PaCO_2$ may actually decrease because of hyperventilation. So the drive to the central control areas in the medulla is not due to decreased PaO_2 or increased $PaCO_2$. It is also not due to decreased pH. There are so-called proprioceptors in muscles and tendons that are turned on by movements of the joints and that signal the medullary centers to increase breathing. But the responses to these receptors are rather puny and it is not likely that they are responsible for the hyperpnea of exercise. There are also chemoreceptors in skeletal muscle that respond to lactate and other metabolic products and could conceivably be involved in exercise hyperpnea. But the evidence for their importance is weak.

Another possibility is "central command", meaning that the cerebral cortex somehow directs the medullary centers to control ventilation according to demand or according to how intensely it is directing the exercising muscles to contract. In favor of this mechanism is the fact that increased breathing often begins very early in exercise or even before exercise begins.

An interesting observation is that even during the most intense and prolonged exercise possible for a given person, that person can always voluntarily breathe harder than the amount of exercise demands. So it is not the ability to increase alveolar ventilation that limits oxygen delivery to exercising muscle. Rather it is the ability of the circulatory system to deliver blood that limits oxygen delivery.

Part 5: Pulmonary Reflexes

Hering-Breuer Reflexes (discovered in 1868 by Hering and Breuer)

The tracheobronchial tree has stretch receptors that sense hyperinflation of the lungs and send a signal to the brain stem centers (*via* the vagus) to stop inspiring. The receptors are called slowly adapting stretch receptors since with maintained overinflation their firing rate subsides only very slowly. In adults, this reflex is thought to protect the lungs against overinflation; it is thought not to have any role in normal eupnea since it doesn't kick in until the lungs are inflated far beyond a normal tidal volume. In infants, it may contribute to limitation of tidal volume during normal breathing and increase breathing frequency. There is also a Hering-Breuer deflation reflex which apparently signals the medullary centers to stop actively exhaling if lung volume becomes excessively low.

It seems apparent that these reflexes must be overridden during intense exercise in order to obtain the necessary increases in tidal volume.

Irritant Receptors

Located between airway epithelial cells, these receptors sense noxious stuff such as cigarette smoke, inhaled dust, ether, and ammonia. They also respond to excessive serotonin, bradykinin, prostaglandins, and histamine. Thus, they are probably stimulated during inflammation. Sensory information travels in the vagus to the NTS. The reflex response is bronchoconstriction and hyperpnea. Coughing and sneezing also result from stimulation of irritant receptors in the upper airways including the nose and nasopharynx. The response to histamine might be important in the bronchoconstriction of asthma. The irritant receptors are rapidly adapting compared to the slowly adapting receptors involved in the Hering-Breuer reflexes.

J Receptors

J is for juxtacapillary. These receptors are in the alveolar walls very near alveolar capillaries. They are apparently stimulated by capillary engorgement and pulmonary edema. The reflex responses include rapid, shallow breathing, bronchoconstriction, and increased secretion of mucus into the airways. These receptors may be involved in the feelings of dyspnea in left heart failure.

Part 6: Complex Pulmonary Activities

There are many reflexes and other activities that involve airflow and temporary interruption of normal breathing. The following is a partial list of these. No attempt is made here to describe the reflex pathways.

- Sighing and yawning
  These occasional activities are thought to help reverse the normal tendency for alveolar collapse (atelectasis).

- Coughing and sneezing
- Swallowing, vomiting, and retching
- Speaking, laughing, singing, whistling, grunting, and playing wind instruments

Part 7: What Can Go Wrong?

Topic: Periodic Breathing Patterns

Cheyne-Stokes Breathing

The most common type of periodic breathing is called Cheyne-Stokes breathing It is characterized by regular periods of waxing and then waning tidal volume that last about 40 to 60 seconds. These periods are separated from each other by shorter periods of apnea. This abnormal breathing pattern sometimes occurs in patients with congestive heart failure, strokes, brain tumors, and carbon monoxide poisoning. It also sometimes occurs in normal people while sleeping at high altitude. The mechanism and importance of Cheyne-Stokes breathing are not well understood.

Biot's Breathing

Biot's breathing is characterized by periods of regular breathing separated by periods of apnea. It is sometimes seen in patients with increased intracranial pressure or meningitis. It is caused by damage to the medulla oblongata.

Kussmahl Breathing

Kussmahl breathing consists of regular, very deep breathing at normal or subnormal frequency. It occurs during severe metabolic acidosis, especially the ketoacidosis of diabetes.

Central Sleep Apnea

Central sleep apnea is characterized by periodic absence of breathing effort throughout sleep. Apparently this disorder is caused by some defect in medullary control.

Obstructive Sleep Apnea

In obstructive sleep apnea respiratory efforts continue but actual breathing periodically stops because of upper airway obstruction. Obstructive sleep apnea is far more common than central sleep apnea. There is also a form of the disorder called complex (or mixed) sleep apnea that combines the features of pure central and pure obstructive sleep apnea.

Ondine's Curse

This is an extremely rare form of central sleep apnea, also known as congenital central hypoventilation syndrome. The apneic periods may be very long or even continuous during sleep, but can be absent or brief while awake. Obviously, without a mechanical respirator while sleeping, these patients die early on. They can, however, successfully breathe voluntarily while awake.

[Once upon a time there was a sea nymph who married a regular man named Hans. Her name was Ondine. Hans was unfaithful and she retaliated with a curse that included the stipulation that he could breathe by voluntary effort but not automatically. So if Hans ever fell asleep he would die. Eventually, in the fairy tale, he did.]

Chapter 12

Regulation of Acid-Base Balance

Part 1: A Brief Primer

Topic 1: Pure Water

Pure water is almost entirely H_2O, but at any instant about one in every 1.8 billion water molecules is dissociated as H^+ and OH^-. H^+ ions are identical to protons. Some of the protons combine with another water molecule to form the hydronium ion (H_3O^+), but we can ignore the distinction between H^+ and H_3O^+ and regard them all as hydrogen ions. A neutral solution is one in which the concentration of H^+ equals the concentration of OH^-. Pure water is always neutral. At $20°$ C the concentration of both H^+ and OH^- in pure water is 1.0×10^{-7} moles/liter, which is the same as 100 nanomolar (nM). At body temperature ($37°$ C) there is somewhat more dissociation of water and the concentration of both H^+ and OH^- at neutrality is 158 nM.

Topic 2: Acids and Bases

An acid is a chemical that releases a proton when it dissolves in water. Release of the proton is by ionization. The proton, of course, has a positive charge. The chemical that released the proton then has a negative charge.

Strong acid: A strong acid is one that ionizes completely (or nearly so) in solution. A simple example is hydrochloric acid, $HCl \rightarrow H^+ + Cl^-$.

Weak acid: A weak acid is one that only partially ionizes in solution and the reaction is reversible. A relevant example is carbonic acid, $H_2CO_3 \leftrightarrow H^+ + HCO_3^-$. Many proteins and phosphate compounds are also weak acids. A very important weak acid is hemoglobin.

A base (or alkali) is a chemical substance that takes up a proton when it dissolves in water. Many bases act by releasing a hydroxyl ion (OH^-) rather than by directly binding a proton. But when hydroxyl ions are released in an aqueous solution they combine with hydrogen ions to form water.

Strong base: A strong base is one that completely ionizes in solution. A good example is $NaOH \rightarrow Na^+ + OH^-$.

Weak base: A weak base is one that takes up protons reversibly to form an equilibrium distribution of protons, acid, and base. A good example is ammonia, NH_3. In aqueous solution it binds protons reversibly to form ammonium ions, $NH_3 + H^+ \leftrightarrow NH_4^+$.

When an acid is added to pure water the H^+ concentration rises and the OH^- concentration falls equally. The opposite happens when a base is added. When the H^+ concentration rises, we say that the acidity has increased; when it falls we say that the acidity has decreased (or the alkalinity has increased).

[Note: Just how much the H^+ and OH^- concentrations change when given amounts of weak acids or weak bases are added to pure water (or to blood) does not have a simple explanation. A theory for this has been developed by P.A. Stuart (*How to Understand Acid-Base*, 1981) but it is beyond the scope of this book.]

There are many acids and bases in body fluids. Ordinarily they balance each other such that the H^+ concentration in arterial blood plasma and other extracellular spaces ranges between about 35 and 45 nM, and averages 40 nM.

It is important that the H^+ concentration in blood not get too high or too low. Most enzymes are sensitive to the concentration of H^+; some are very sensitive and will not function properly with abnormal acidity. This is also true of membrane transporters and channels. The body has ways of correcting for abnormalities in acid/base balance. The compensatory mechanisms involve the respiratory system and the renal system.

Topic 3: Buffers

A buffer is a chemical that can reversibly combine with protons or release protons depending on acidity, thereby attenuating their buildup or decline in solution. A buffer can be a weak acid or a weak base. Buffers in blood help to prevent large swings in acidity when either acids or bases are added.

Buffering power: The amount of an added acid or base required to change the pH of a solution (such as blood plasma) one pH unit is called the buffering power of that solution.

By far the most important buffer system in blood plasma is the carbon dioxide/bicarbonate system (CO_2/HCO_3^-). It depends on the familiar CO_2 hydration reaction:

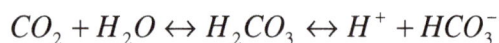

$$CO_2 + H_2O \leftrightarrow H_2CO_3 \leftrightarrow H^+ + HCO_3^-$$

It is sometimes useful to ignore the intermediate carbonic acid (H_2CO_3) and simply write

$$CO_2 + H_2O \leftrightarrow H^+ + HCO_3^-$$

We will call this the condensed CO_2 hydration reaction. Notice that when the H^+ concentration rises this reaction moves to the left, thereby removing some of the extra H^+ and forming more CO_2. When H^+ concentration falls the reaction goes to the right which generates more H^+ and uses up CO_2.

There are other buffers in blood plasma including plasma proteins and phosphates, but the CO_2/bicarbonate buffer system is by far the most important. In red cells hemoglobin is a tremendously important buffer.

Topic 4: An Important Feature of CO_2 as an Acid and CO_2/HCO_3^- as a Buffer System

CO_2 is not really an acid itself, but it behaves like an acid because it is converted to carbonic acid (H_2CO_3) in the CO_2 hydration reaction. So we can consider CO_2 to be an acid and this is implicit in the condensed CO_2 hydration reaction. CO_2 is a very remarkable acid since its partial pressure in arterial blood is regulated by pulmonary ventilation to a nearly constant value, normally about 40 mmHg (equivalent to a concentration of about 1.2 mM). Thus, if the H^+ concentration in blood rises as a result of non-respiratory activity, such as release of lactic acid from exercising muscle by anaerobic metabolism, the CO_2 hydration reaction goes to the left, generating CO_2. But this extra CO_2 is automatically blown off due to increased alveolar ventilation and the $PaCO_2$ remains essentially constant. The virtue of this is that there is no buildup of CO_2 and, therefore, the reaction rate is not slowed by mass action. The only thing limiting the disposal of excess protons in blood is the bicarbonate concentration.

Topic 5: The pH Scale

So far we have been using nM as the unit of H^+ concentration. Unfortunately, the unit of acidity customarily used is the pH unit (devised by Sorensen in 1909). The pH is defined as follows:

$$pH = \log \frac{1}{[H^+]}$$

$\log$ *is to the base* 10

$[H^+]$ *is molar hydrogen ion* (*proton*) *concentration*

This is the same as :

$$pH = -\log[H^+]$$

There may be some justification for using a logarithmic scale in certain chemistry applications since it compresses a wide range of concentration values into manageable numbers. But, as convincingly explained by Grogono (www.acid-base.com), the pH scale has no virtue in physiology or medicine. It significantly impairs learning and it leads to constant confusion. But we are stuck with it. We must teach acid/base balance using the pH scale since it has become traditional and is universally used in medical practice.

Using the pH scale, neutral pH at 37° C is 6.8. This is calculated as -log (0.000000158). Normal average pH in arterial blood is 7.40, and the normal pH range is about 7.35 to 7.45.

Part 2: The Relationship between the Concentrations of Acid, Base, and Protons

Topic 1: The Henderson Equation

The equilibrium equation for the condensed CO_2 hydration reaction is:

$$Ka = \frac{[HCO_3^-] \times [H^+]}{[CO_2]}$$

Ka is the dissociation constant for the weak acid. It has a value of about 800 nM.

Solving for [H$^+$] we get:

$$[H^+] = Ka \times \frac{[CO_2]}{[HCO_3^-]}$$

The concentration of CO_2 equals its solubility coefficient multiplied by its partial pressure. Therefore:

$$[H^+] = Ka \times \frac{0.03 \times PCO_2}{[HCO_3^-]}$$

This is the Henderson equation. It should be sufficient. But wait. Owing to tradition, we must now deal with logarithms.

Topic 2: The Henderson-Hasselbalch Equation

We take the reciprocal of both sides of the Henderson equation to get:

$$\frac{1}{[H^+]} = \frac{1}{Ka} \times \frac{[HCO_3^-]}{0.03 \times PCO_2}$$

Then we take the log$_{10}$ of both sides to get:

$$pH = pKa + \log \frac{[HCO_3^-]}{0.03 \times PCO_2}$$

pKa = 6.1. This is -log (800 nM)

Therefore:

$$pH = 6.1 + \log \frac{[HCO_3^-]}{0.03 \times PaCO_2}$$

This is the famous Henderson-Hasselbalch equation. It doesn't do anything for us that the simpler Henderson equation does not do, but we're stuck with it.

There are three variables in the Henderson-Hasselbalch equation: pH, [HCO$_3^-$], and PaCO$_2$. If we measure any two of these we can calculate the other one. In clinical arterial blood gas analysis (ABG) pH and PaCO$_2$ are usually measured by electrodes and bicarbonate concentration is automatically calculated by use of the Henderson-Hasselbalch equation.

Using normal values for [HCO$_3^-$] (24 mM) and PaCO$_2$, (40 mmHg), the Henderson-Hasselbalch equation becomes:

$$pH = 6.1 + \log \frac{24}{1.2} = 6.1 + \log(20) = 7.4$$

As long as the ratio [HCO$_3^-$] / [CO$_2$] is 20, the pH will be 7.4. For example, if the CO$_2$ concentration rises but the bicarbonate concentration rises proportionately, the pH will still be 7.4. The concentration of HCO$_3^-$ is determined mainly by the kidneys while the concentration of CO$_2$ is determined by alveolar ventilation.

Part 3: Abnormalities of Arterial Acidity

Topic 1: The Problems

There are four primary abnormalities of arterial pH. These are respiratory acidosis, respiratory alkalosis, metabolic acidosis, and metabolic alkalosis.

Respiratory Acidosis and Alkalosis

Respiratory acidosis is caused by increased $PaCO_2$ due to hypoventilation. The CO_2 hydration reaction is driven to the right and, consequently, plasma $[HCO_3^-]$ is increased. Respiratory acidosis can result acutely from voluntary breath holding as in underwater swimming, from various drugs that depress the respiratory center, or chronically from a variety of pulmonary diseases that involve reduced alveolar ventilation. A more complete list of causes is included at the end of this chapter.

Respiratory alkalosis is caused by reduced $PaCO_2$ due to hyperventilation. The bicarbonate concentration is low. An interesting cause can be hypoxemia which induces hyperventilation by stimulating the carotid bodies. This is common, for example, at high altitudes. Other causes include psychogenic hyperventilation and severe fever.

Metabolic Acidosis and Alkalosis

Metabolic acidosis is acidosis that is caused by anything other than hypoventilation. It is characterized by decreased plasma bicarbonate concentration. Metabolic acidosis includes lactic acidosis that can occur during intense and prolonged exercise or during circulatory shock. It also includes the ketoacidosis of diabetes. Renal causes include various disorders that result in reduced ability to acidify the urine. The most important gastrointestinal cause is diarrhea since colonic fluid is alkaline. Losing a lot of base has the same effect on arterial pH as gaining a lot of acid. In addition, ingesting excessive amounts of aspirin (acetyl salicylic acid) can lead to metabolic acidosis.

Metabolic alkalosis is alkalosis caused by anything other than hyperventilation. It is characterized by increased plasma $[HCO_3^-]$. Causes include vomiting (since the lost gastric juice is highly acidic), and aggressive antacid therapy.

Mixed Acid/Base Disturbances

It often happens that a respiratory acid/base imbalance coexists with a metabolic acid/base disturbance. For example, a patient with emphysema who has respiratory acidosis (due to CO_2 retention) will probably also be hypoxemic. The hypoxemia is likely to lead to increased anaerobic metabolism is tissues with resulting lactic acidosis. Another example is a patient with anxiety-related respiratory alkalosis who could also happen to have a gastric problem leading to a lot of antacid ingestion. Hyperventilation plus antacids would lead to a mixed respiratory/renal alkalosis. There might also be a patient who tends to be acidotic because of diarrhea, but also tends to be alkalotic because of hyperventilation.

Topic 2: The Compensations

Changes in alveolar ventilation can partially compensate for a metabolic acid/base disturbance (*i.e.* bring pH back toward normal). Changes in H^+ or HCO_3^- excretion by the kidneys can partially compensate for a respiratory acid/base disturbance. Respiratory compensation is very prompt while renal compensation is slower (hours to days). Respiratory compensation adjusts the $PaCO_2$ term in the Henderson-Hasselbalch equation, while renal compensation adjusts the $[HCO_3^-]$ term.

Renal Compensation for Respiratory Acidosis

Respiratory acidosis is characterized by high plasma $[HCO_3^-]$. The kidneys can adjust the amount of H^+ and the amount of bicarbonate that are eliminated in the urine. They can also adjust the amount of new bicarbonate that is made in distal tubules and transported into blood. The kidneys perform these adjustments in response to the pH of arterial blood. The renal tubular transport mechanisms that perform these adjustments will not be described here.

In respiratory acidosis the kidneys excrete more H^+ and salvage some bicarbonate. An important fraction of excreted H^+ is in the form of ammonium ions, NH^+. The result is a further elevation of plasma $[HCO_3^-]$. This returns arterial pH back up toward normal.

Actually, normal pH cannot be reached and compensation is always incomplete. If compensation were complete there would no longer be any signal to continue the respiratory compensation, so complete compensation is impossible.

Renal Compensation for Respiratory Alkalosis

Respiratory alkalosis is characterized by low plasma [HCO_3^-]. Renal compensation is just the opposite of renal compensation for respiratory acidosis. Plasma [HCO_3^-] is further decreased and arterial pH is returned toward normal.

Respiratory Compensation for Metabolic Acidosis

Metabolic acidosis is characterized by low plasma [HCO_3^-]. The respiratory system responds by increasing alveolar ventilation and, thereby, reducing $PaCO_2$. This returns the [HCO_3^-]/$PaCO_2$ ratio toward normal and, therefore, returns arterial pH toward normal.

The signal that promotes compensation is, of course, low arterial pH. The carotid bodies are the main receptors. The ventilatory response is quite

prompt. There is probably a relatively slow and minor response *via* the central chemoreceptors.

Respiratory Compensation for Metabolic Alkalosis

Metabolic alkalosis is characterized by high plasma [HCO_3^-]. The signal for compensation is high arterial pH and, again, the carotid bodies are the main receptors. The result is alveolar hypoventilation with consequent increase in $PaCO_2$. Therefore, the HCO_3^-/$PaCO_2$ ratio is reduced and pH is returned toward normal.

Renal Compensation for <u>Metabolic</u> Acidosis or Alkalosis

As long as the renal tubular transporters involved in H^+ and bicarbonate movements are functioning properly, the kidneys can help compensate for metabolic acid/base imbalances (caused for example by vomiting or diarrhea) in the same ways that they compensate for respiratory acid/base imbalances.

Part 4: Davenport Diagrams

The above information concerning primary disturbances and compensations can be visualized and, therefore, remembered by using a graphical analysis. The most common graphical analysis was developed by Davenport (H.W. Davenport, *The ABC of Acid-Base Chemistry, 6th Ed.*, 1974).

Topic 1: Simple Metabolic Acid-Base Disturbance

Figure 1
We can easily solve the Henderson-Hasselbalch equation for bicarbonate concentration:

$$[HCO_3^-] = 0.03 \times PCO_2^{(pH-6.1)}$$

Then we plot [HCO_3^-] as a function of pH. The result is shown in Figure 1 which is called a Davenport diagram. This figure illustrates <u>metabolic</u> acidosis and alkalosis at a constant $PaCO_2$ of 40 mmHg.

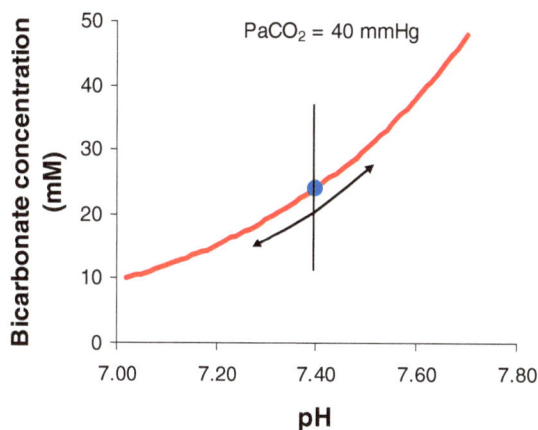

Figure 1. This is a Davenport diagram showing how bicarbonate concentration changes as a result of changing pH by adding acid or base to blood. PCO_2 is constant at a normal value of 40 mmHg. Adding non-bicarbonate acid or base causes <u>metabolic</u> acidosis or alkalosis respectively (indicated by the arrows). Acidosis is to the left of the vertical line, alkalosis is to the right.

As pH decreases in metabolic acidosis, [HCO_3^-] also decreases and the opposite happens when pH increases in metabolic alkalosis.

Topic 2: Respiratory Acid-Base Disturbance

Figure 2

The next Davenport diagram, Figure 2, adds what happens with <u>respiratory</u> acidosis (PCO_2 = 60 or 80 mmHg) and alkalosis (PCO_2 = 20 mmHg).

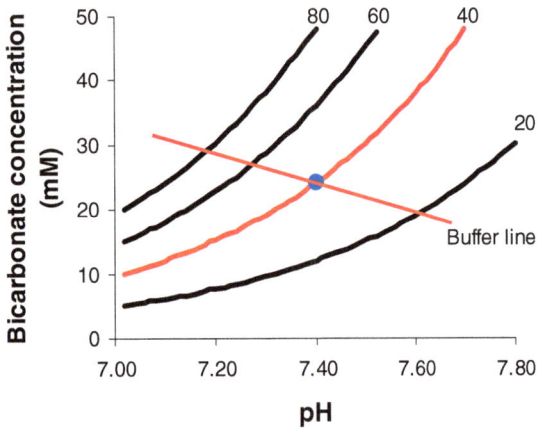

Figure 2. This Davenport diagram shows the effect of decreased $PaCO_2$ due to hyperventilation (respiratory alkalosis) or increased $PaCO_2$ due to hypoventilation (respiratory acidosis). The numbers at the end of each curve represent $PaCO_2$ in mmHg. The straight line is called the <u>buffer line</u>.

The curved lines show [HCO_3^-] as a function of pH at various values for $PaCO_2$, plotted according to the Henderson-Hasselbalch equation. The straight line is called the <u>buffer line</u>. It shows what happens to pH and [HCO_3^-] when $PaCO_2$ is changed. At any given $PaCO_2$, the system must operate at the point where the buffer line intersects the curved bicarbonate *vs.* pH line.

The buffer line would be essentially flat if there were no non-bicarbonate buffers since then, with elevation of $PaCO_2$, only a minute amount of H^+ and HCO_3^- could be generated from the CO_2 hydration reaction. This reaction is normally kept going enough to generate a lot of HCO_3^- because of H^+ uptake by non-bicarbonate buffers, mainly hemoglobin and phosphates.

Topic 3: The Buffer Line Shifts When Acid or Base is Added

Figure 3

The next Davenport diagram shows effects of metabolic acidosis and alkalosis on the buffer line.

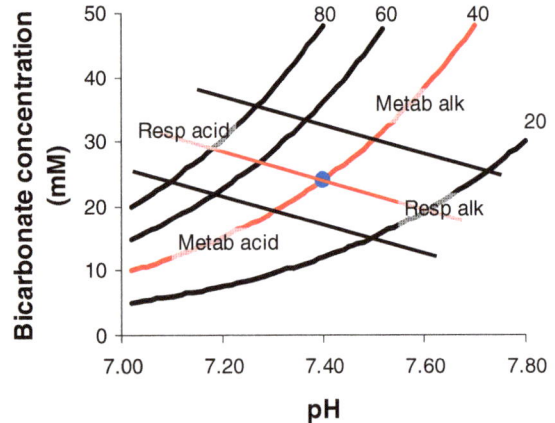

Figure 3. This Davenport diagram adds two more buffer lines, one for a primary metabolic acidosis (lower line) and one for a primary metabolic alkalosis (upper line).

In Figure 3, the lowest buffer line shows how the blood buffers CO_2 after it has undergone metabolic acidosis (initially to pH 7.3 at PCO_2 = 40 mmHg). The top buffer line shows how the system buffers CO_2 after it has undergone metabolic alkalosis (initially to pH 7.5 at PCO_2 = 40 mmHg). The buffer lines parallel each other. Figure 3 illustrates the following characteristics of acidosis and alkalosis:

Type	[HCO_3^-]
Respiratory acidosis	High
Metabolic acidosis	Low
Respiratory alkalosis	Low
Metabolic alkalosis	High

These simple criteria are useful for an initial diagnosis. The situation can be more complex, however, if both a respiratory and a metabolic disturbance are present together (mixed acid/base imbalance).

Topic 4: Use of Davenport Diagrams for Visualizing Primary Problems and Compensations

Figure 4

This is a Davenport diagram that shows the compensations in addition to the primary problems.

- The green arrow shows a pure respiratory acidosis (first segment) followed by partial renal compensation (second segment). The primary cause (hypoventilation) raises [HCO$_3$] as it lowers pH; renal compensation raises [HCO$_3$] further, thereby increasing pH.
- The pink arrow represents pure metabolic alkalosis (persistent vomiting, too much antacid, etc.) followed by respiratory compensation (hypoventilation). The [HCO$_3$] increases during both phases.
- The brown arrow is for primary metabolic acidosis (*e.g.* diabetic ketoacidosis) followed by respiratory compensation.
- The blue arrow represents primary respiratory alkalosis followed by renal compensation.

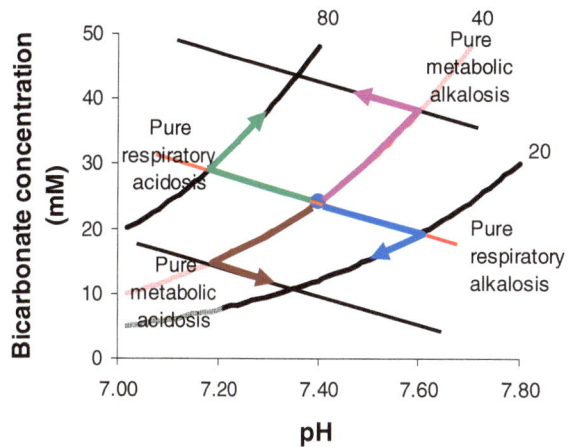

Figure 4. This Davenport diagram includes arrows showing primary acid/base imbalances (first segment of each arrow) and compensations (second segment of each arrow). See text for explanations.

Part 5: Assessing the Metabolic Contribution to an Acid/Base Imbalance

Topic 1: Base Excess

Figure 5

This is the same as Figure 4 but also illustrates the concept of base excess. First look at the green arrow for respiratory acidosis. After renal compensation, the pH is back to about 7.3 and the bicarbonate concentration is about 38 mM. The bicarbonate concentration is about 10 mM greater than it would have been with a pure respiratory acidosis to pH 7.3. The renal compensation has created a base excess (BE) of about 10 mM. In Figure 5 the base excess is indicated by the vertical arrow. The value for base excess provides an estimate of how much renal compensation there has been.

Note that if there had initially been a respiratory acidosis to pH 7.3 and there had been no compensation, the base excess would have been zero. Normal values for base excess range between ± 2 mM.

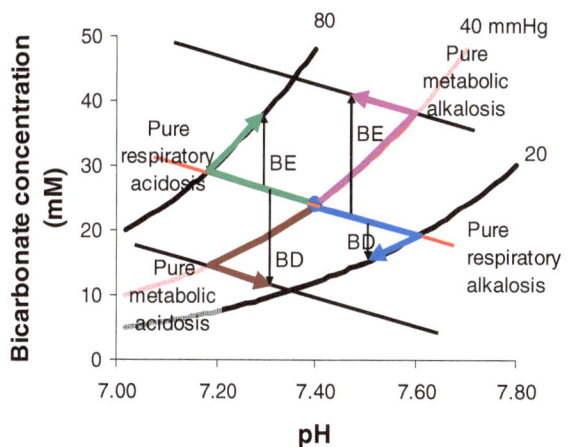

Figure 5. This Davenport diagram shows how the base excess or base deficit can be determined. The method assumes that the buffer lines parallel each other which may not actually be the case.

Next consider the pink arrow for metabolic alkalosis with compensation. The up arrow connecting the normal buffer line with the final $[HCO_3^-]$/pH point represents a base excess of about 18 mM. In this case, the base excess results entirely from the primary metabolic alkalosis. So, again, base excess is a measure of the metabolic (*i.e.* non-respiratory) component of the problem.

The brown arrow for compensated metabolic acidosis ends at a $[HCO_3^-]$ of about 12 mM. This is about 15 mM less than it would be if the pH were the same but there were no metabolic acidosis (down arrow). This is called a <u>base deficit</u> (BD). It is also known as a <u>negative base excess</u>. The base deficit in metabolic acidosis can be helpful clinically for estimating how much bicarbonate to use in treatment.

The blue arrow for respiratory alkalosis with compensation also ends at a base deficit.

[The official definition of a base excess or base deficit is the amount of HCl or NaOH that would be required to titrate a sample of blood plasma back to pH 7.4 after it had already been equilibrated with a PCO_2 of 40 mmHg at 37°C. It is a little hard to prove this, but the vertical distance between parallel buffer lines on a Davenport diagram is equivalent to this definition.]

Davenport diagrams are not ordinarily used clinically for determining base excess or deficit. Instead, equations developed by Siggaard-Andersen for estimating base excess are built right into the blood gas analyzers. These instruments do not all use the same variation of the Siggaard-Andersen equations and, consequently, their outputs can vary appreciably. Thus, it is important for each hospital to have its own standards.

Topic 2: Anion Gap

A simpler method for estimating the magnitude of non-respiratory involvement in metabolic acidosis involves comparing the summed concentrations of the major cations in blood plasma to that of the major anions. Ordinarily:

$$[Na^+] + [K^+] - [Cl^-] - [HCO_3^-] \approx 15 \text{ mEq/liter}$$

This difference is called the anion gap. Of course there must actually be the same total concentration of positive charges as there are negative charges (*i.e.* there must be electroneutrality). The normal anion gap of about 15 is due to various unmeasured

anions such as plasma proteins and phosphates. In metabolic acidosis the anion gap can be much greater than this due to the presence of unmeasured lactate, ketoacids, *etc.*

Sometimes K^+ is not bothered with for calculating anion gap. In this case the normal value is roughly 11 mEq/liter.

Optional:
But What If We Didn't Bother With Logarithms?

Let's take the Henderson equation:

$$[H^+] = Ka \times \frac{[CO_2]}{[HCO_3^-]}$$

Solving for HCO_3^- we get:

$$[HCO_3^-] = Ka \times \frac{[CO_2]}{[H^+]}$$

We know that Ka = 800 nM and $[CO_2] = 0.03 \times PaCO_2$ mM

Now we plot $[HCO_3^-]$ as a function of $[H^+]$:

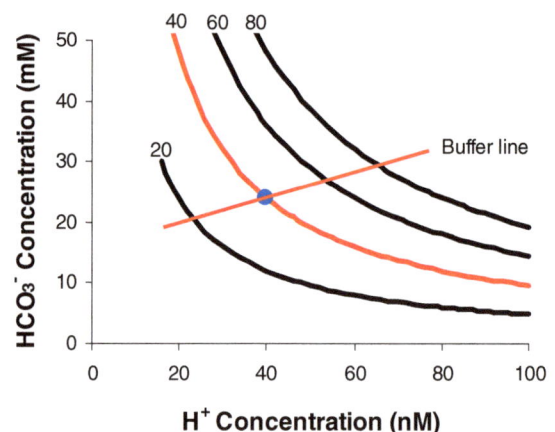

This is a Davenport diagram without the foolishness of logs. All of the same developments that we did with regular Davenport diagrams could be pursued with logless diagrams, but there is no need to bother.

Part 6: What Can Go Wrong?

Topic: Some Major Causes of Acid-Base Disturbances

Respiratory Acidosis:
Restrictive Pulmonary Disorders
    Neuromuscular
- Poliomyelitis
- Amyotrophic lateral sclerosis
- Multiple sclerosis
- Myasthenia gravis
- Periodic paralysis

    Other
- Diffuse Interstitial pulmonary fibrosis
- Myxedema
- Scleroderma
- Extreme obesity
- Kyphoscoliosis
- Pneumothorax

Obstructive Pulmonary Disorders
- COPD (emphysema, chronic bronchitis)
- Asthma

Depression of Respiratory Center
- Drugs (opiates, sedatives, alcohol, anesthetics)
- Central sleep apnea

Localized Airway Obstruction
- Obstructive sleep apnea
- Laryngospasm
- Aspiration of foreign object

Others
- ARDS (adult/acute respiratory distress syndrome)
- Infant respiratory distress syndrome
- Pulmonary edema
- Pneumonia

Respiratory Alkalosis
Voluntary or anxiety-related hyperventilation
Fever
Hypoxemia (*e.g.* at high altitude)

Metabolic Acidosis
Renal failure
Various renal tubular disorders of acid secretion or bicarbonate retention
Lactic acidosis (circulatory shock)
Ketoacidosis (diabetes)
Salicylate poisoning
Diarrhea

Metabolic Alkalosis
Vomiting
Antacid therapy
Loop or thiazide diuretics
Mineralocorticoid (aldosterone) excess
Hypercalcemia
Hypokalemia

Chapter 13

Air Processing

Warming and Humidifying
As inhaled air passes over the epithelium of the upper airways, its temperature and water vapor pressure equilibrate with those of blood. This results in an inhaled air temperature of 37° C and a water partial pressure of 47 mmHg. During nose breathing, air conditioning is nearly completed in the nose and pharynx. During mouth breathing, there is some delay, but apparently without adverse consequences.

Inspired air may contain dust, pollen, fungal spores, bacteria, viruses, asbestos, silica, toxic chemicals, and products of combustion. In addition, food particles and bacteria are sometimes accidentally aspirated into the airways. How does the pulmonary system deal with these contaminants?

Filtration
Filtration is especially effective during nose breathing. The nasal hairs over the extensive surface area of the nasal septum and turbinates retain most inhaled particles with diameters greater than about 5-10 μm. These particles become entrapped in the mucus that covers the nasal mucosa, which is subsequently blown out or sucked in.

Capture by Mucus along the Airways
Many particles that escape nasal filtration collide with the mucus that coats the airways and become entrapped in it. The mucus is secreted by goblet cells in the epithelium and by mucous glands in the submucosa. Collision of particles with mucus is due to diffusion, Brownian motion, gravity, and linear inertial movement of the particles at bends and bifurcations of the airway system. For example, the sudden bend at the nasopharynx results in mucus capture of many particles along the posterior pharyngeal surface. Mucus at the carina and the numerous bronchiole branch points also captures many foreign particles. Sedimentation onto the mucus layer due to gravity plays a larger role in the smaller airways where the velocity of airflow is very low. The result is removal of almost all particles with diameters greater than about 2 μm before the alveoli are reached.

Particles less than about 0.5 μm in diameter tend to form a stable suspension in air (an aerosol). Most of these very tiny particles are not trapped by mucus, but are simply breathed out.

Removal of Filtered and Mucus-Captured Particles

Coughing and Sneezing
Expiratory airflow velocity during coughing and sneezing can approach the speed of sound. These reflexes expel much of the mucus-entrapped particles from the upper airways.

The Mucociliary Escalator
Figure 1
The airways, all the way down to the terminal bronchioles, have a ciliated epithelium. The cilia beat in a way that propels the overlying layer of gelatinous mucus, with entrapped foreign particles, toward the mouth. The layer of gelatinous mucus rides on a serous subphase (pericilliary layer) as shown in Figure 1.

The serous subphase is not gelated; it is a salt solution secreted mainly by the serous cells of the epithelium. The cilia beat at a frequency of as much as 1300 per minute. By this means, airway mucus is propelled toward the mouth at a velocity of roughly 0.5 mm/min in small airways and as much as 20 mm/min in the trachea. From the mouth, airway mucus (with entrapped foreign particles) is normally swallowed, blown, coughed, or spitted. Patients who cannot do these maneuvers must be assisted by suction.

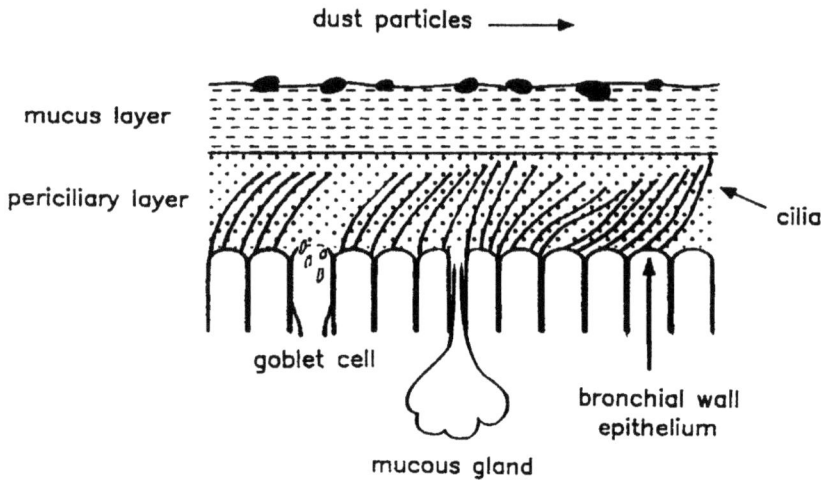

Figure 1. The mucociliary escalator. The ciliated epithelium of airways is coated by a fluid layer that is about 5-10 μm thick. The innermost part of this coating is a highly viscous mucus gel. It rides over a serous (watery) subphase sometimes called the pericilliary layer. Inhaled particles are trapped in the mucus layer as described in the text. There are about 250 cilia per epithelial cell and they are about 5-7 μm long. The cilia beat at a frequency up to 1300/min. During their forward stroke, their tips touch the mucus layer, moving it toward the mouth. During their backstroke, their tips move entirely within the serous layer. Waves of activity seem to pass over extended regions of epithelium in a highly coordinated fashion. From G. Sant'Ambrogio and F.B. Sant'Ambrogio, Mechanics of Breathing: Statics, in *The Medical Physiology and Biophysics Syllabus*, UTMB, 1998.

The Role of Alveolar Macrophages in Handling Contaminants

Alveolar macrophages are the creatures of the pulmonary deep. They prowl the alveoli in search of stuff to eat. They ingest any particles that have escaped filtration and mucus entrapment in the airways above. Some particles, including bacteria, are digested by macrophagic lysosomes. Other kinds of particles such as silica cannot be digested and simply accumulate in the macrophages, which eventually die (lifetime of a few weeks) and then migrate onto the mucociliary escalator *via* the pores of Kohn. Some particle-laden alveolar macrophages migrate through the alveolar epithelium and are carried away in lymph. [Alveolar macrophages are also importantly involved in pulmonary immune and inflammatory responses, but details on this topic are beyond the scope of this book.]

Other Processes for Handling Foreign Particles

Some particles cross the alveolar epithelium; some of these are phagocytized in the interstitial space or blood, while others simply enter the lymphatics. Some bacteria are destroyed by lysozymes, lactoferrin, and other enzymes derived from leucocytes and submucosal gland cells. Alpha$_1$ antitrypsin helps to inactivate proteolytic enzymes released from dead bacteria in the alveoli. Interferon α probably helps to kill viruses in the alveoli. Lastly, antibody-mediated and cell-mediated immunological responses are thought to inactivate many contaminants.

Chapter 14

Exercise

This chapter will focus on relatively prolonged, continuous, rhythmic exercise done at a reasonably constant intensity level. During the sustained period, ATP production is mostly due to oxidative phosphorylation rather than anaerobic glycolysis. Consequently, this sort of exertion is commonly called <u>aerobic</u> exercise. Examples include running, walking, swimming, bicycling, *etc*. On the other hand, relatively brief bursts of exertion mainly utilize creatine phosphate and anaerobic glycolysis for generating ATP and are often called <u>anaerobic</u> exercise. Examples include weight lifting and sprinting.

Topic 1: Time Course for Effect of Exercise on Pulmonary Ventilation

Figure 1

Everybody knows that as we exercise harder we breathe harder. We breathe deeper and faster, and this brings in more oxygen and blows off more carbon dioxide. A typical time course for this effect is illustrated in Figure 1 for an exercise intensity that is mild to moderate and is steady.

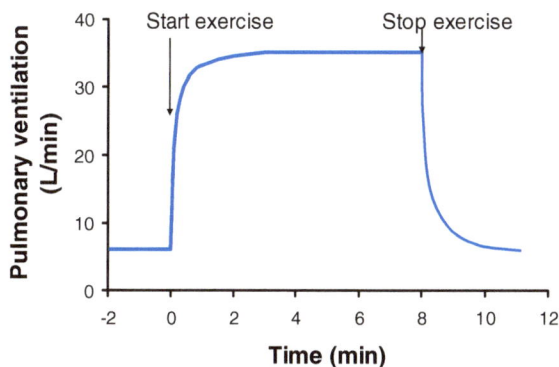

Figure 1. Total pulmonary ventilation as a function of time during exercise of moderate intensity. The abrupt changes at start and end are thought to be due mainly to central command. [Note: all charts in this chapter are idealized representations of the data, which actually have considerable scatter.]

The sudden initial increase in pulmonary ventilation, $\dot{V}_E$, is usually thought to be mainly a <u>central command</u> effect, similar to the one for increasing cardiac output during exercise. According to this theory, when the cerebral cortex induces skeletal muscle to exercise, it simultaneously activates cardiovascular and respiratory centers in the medulla.

There is then a gradual rise in $\dot{V}_E$ that reaches a plateau. The height of this plateau (*i.e.* steady-state $\dot{V}_E$) depends on the intensity of exercise; in fact the two are matched amazingly well. We don't know how this matching works, as was discussed in Chapter 11, Part 4. Over the low exercise intensity range, increased $\dot{V}_E$ is mainly due to increased tidal volume. As exercise intensity increases further, the rise in $\dot{V}_E$ is increasingly dependent on breathing frequency.

Topic 2: Time Course for Effect of Exercise on Oxygen Consumption, $\dot{V}O_2$

Figure 2

$\dot{V}O_2$ increases during steady exercise with a time course similar to that of $\dot{V}_E$, except that the sudden initial increase and sudden final decrease are missing

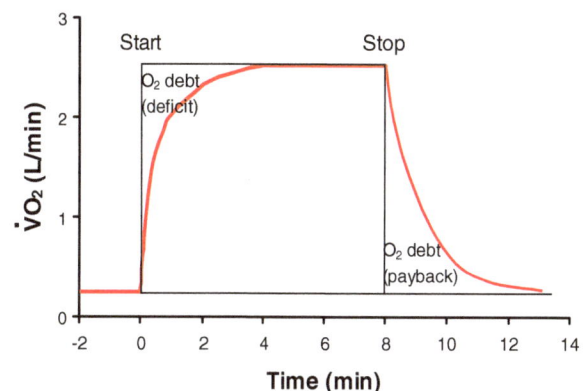

Figure 2. Rate of oxygen consumption, $\dot{V}O_2$ (red curve), during and following a bout of moderate intensity exercise.

The top horizontal line in Figure 1 estimates the rate of oxygen utilization necessary if all the ATP utilized to perform the exercise were immediately replenished by oxidative phosphorylation only. Note that during the first few minutes $\dot{V}O_2$ rises gradually until a plateau is reached. During the plateau, oxidative phosphorylation keeps up with ATP demand. But at first it doesn't. Instead, ATP is generated from creatine phosphate (CP) by the following reaction:

$$ADP + CP \rightarrow ATP + C$$

This reaction is so fast and the supply of CP so abundant in muscle mitochondria that during exercise of moderate intensity the concentration of ATP is maintained near resting level for a considerable length of time.

The gradual early rise in $\dot{V}O_2$ continues until the rate of oxidative phosphorylation catches up to meet the task. Anaerobic glycolysis assists in generating ATP during this period.

The area surrounded by the vertical and horizontal lines at start and the rising $\dot{V}O_2$ curve represents the additional amount of O_2 that would have been needed during this time if all ATP generation had been accomplished by oxidative phosphorylation. This amount of O_2 is called the oxygen debt (sometimes called the oxygen deficit); it will have to be repaid after exercise stops.

Notice that when exercise abruptly stops, the rate of O_2 consumption only gradually goes back down to baseline. Now, the area enclosed by the lines and the curve is the oxygen payback (often it is still called the O_2 debt). Usually payback is somewhat larger than the original debt; in other words, there is some interest. Oxygen payback is necessary to rebuild CP, ATP, and glycogen stores and, after intense exercise, metabolize excess lactic acid.

Topic 3: Measures of Exercise Intensity

Power
Exercise intensity is often quantified in terms of power output. Power is defined as the rate of work done. Work in Joules is divided by time in seconds to get Watts. Work performed (force x distance) and power can be assessed in some kinds of endurance exercise like stair stepping, inclined treadmill running, or variable-resistance stationary bicycling. In fact, stationary bikes in gyms often

provide a Watts output on the control panel. [An older way of expressing power, which is still often used. is KiloCalories/min.]

Rate of Oxygen Consumption, $\dot{V}O_2$
Figure 3
Instead of power output, the rate of oxygen consumption is often used as a measure of exercise intensity. Figure 3 shows why this is valid. Up to very high exercise intensities, the increase in $\dot{V}O_2$ is nearly linear. Eventually it can't increase any further and a $\dot{V}O_2$ maximum is reached. But in most of the usual range of exercise intensities, $\dot{V}O_2$ can be substituted for Watts. Often, the percent of $\dot{V}O_2$ max for each individual is used since this tends to normalize among people capable of a wide range of maximal exercise intensities.

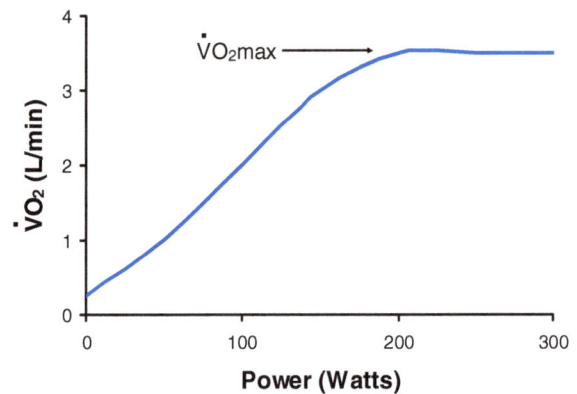

Figure 3. Over a wide range of exercise intensities, almost to $\dot{V}O_2$ max, the relationship between O_2 consumption and power output is nearly linear.

Exercise intensities up to roughly 25% of $\dot{V}O_2$ max are considered mild, from 25% to 60% are moderate, and from 60% to 100% are intense.

Topic 4: The $\dot{V}O_2$ max

Figure 3 again
The rate of O_2 consumption during the steady state (plateau) depends on the intensity of exercise – hardly surprising. The important thing is that there is a high level of intensity at which $\dot{V}O_2$ max cannot rise further. This is called the $\dot{V}O_2$ max. If we try to increase the intensity further, we can't, at least not for long. For short bursts we can increase intensity, relying on CP and anaerobic glycolysis for ATP production. But this

cannot last long. So the intensity of prolonged exercise is limited by $\dot{V}O_2$ max .

[Note: Such studies are often done by progressively increasing exercise intensity as time goes on. This so-called incremental exercise routine suffers scientifically from the fact that two variables, intensity and time, may be simultaneously contributing to the effect, but the method seems to work out alright.]

$\dot{V}O_2$ max varies among individuals. It tends to be relatively fixed for any one person since heredity has a lot to do with its value. However, $\dot{V}O_2$ max can be increased somewhat with endurance training. It declines with aging.

Topic 5: The Anaerobic Threshold

Figure 4
This figure shows that at some exercise intensity prior to $\dot{V}O_2$ max , lactate begins building up in the blood. This is because additional exercise intensity must be energized partly by anaerobic glycolysis, which produces lactic acid. The exercise intensity at which blood lactate has clearly increased is called the <u>anaerobic threshold</u> (AT) or the <u>lactate threshold</u> (LT). Actually, it is not possible to determine accurately just when lactate starts rising, so often some arbitrary value that is obviously above baseline is used as the anaerobic threshold.

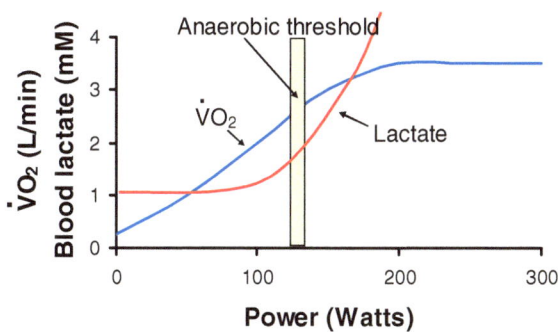

Figure 4. As $\dot{V}O_2$ max is approached, lactate starts building up in the blood and can reach as high as 10 mM or so. The exercise intensity at which blood lactate has clearly risen is called the anaerobic threshold.

Figure 5
Release of lactic acid into the blood following the anaerobic threshold has several consequences:

- Increased lactate concentration as the lactic acid is buffered by bicarbonate.
- Decreased pH.
- Increased pulmonary ventilation, $\dot{V}_E$. This effect is caused mainly by stimulation of peripheral chemoreceptors by the decrease in pH. Extra CO_2 is blown off, thereby attenuating the drop in pH. This is a great example of respiratory compensation for a metabolic acidosis in a normal situation.
- Decreased P_ACO_2 and increased P_AO_2, caused by increased $\dot{V}_E$

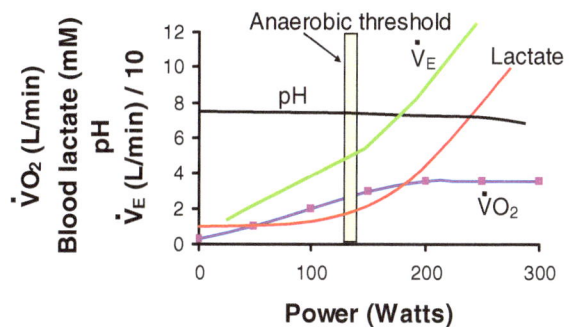

Figure 5. The steep increase in blood lactate concentration following the anaerobic threshold leads to a decrease in blood pH, which promotes an increase in minute volume of breathing, $\dot{V}_E$.

The anaerobic threshold can occur at an exercise intensity anywhere between roughly 50% and 90% of $\dot{V}O_2$ max . Its location depends on heredity and on training. Endurance training can raise the anaerobic threshold. In fact, the measured anaerobic threshold is often used as a measure of fitness and a predictor of performance in endurance athletes.

Sometimes, instead of blood lactate concentration, the anaerobic threshold is estimated as the exercise intensity at which the slope of the $\dot{V}_E$ line increases (in this case it is often called VT). Sometimes the intensity at which alveolar PCO_2 starts to rise is used. Cleary, the value taken for the anaerobic threshold can vary quite a lot depending on the way it is estimated.

Topic 6: Alveolar PO$_2$ and PCO$_2$

Figure 6
This figure shows the effect of progressively increasing exercise intensity on alveolar PO_2 and PCO_2. Note that approximately until the anaerobic

threshold is reached, P_AO_2 and P_ACO_2 both stay remarkably constant. This fact may be very important. If alveolar PO_2 were to go down, increased exercise intensity could be severely limited. An increase in alveolar PO_2 probably would not do much good since Hb would already be saturated, and the increase in ventilation required would unnecessarily increase the energy cost of breathing. So constancy of alveolar PO_2 and PCO_2 is probably optimal.

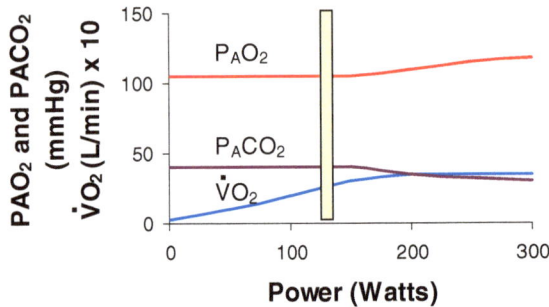

Figure 6. Effect of increasing exercise intensity on alveolar partial pressures of O_2 and CO_2. Oxygen consumption, $\dot{V}O_2$, is shown for comparison. The $\dot{V}O_2$ values are multiplied by 10 so that the same ordinate scale can be used in this chart.

Now, how is this constancy possible? Let's assume that inhaled air FiO_2 remains constant and the respiratory exchange ratio, R, doesn't change much. With those assumptions, there are only two things that determine average alveolar PO_2 and PCO_2. These are the total lung $\dot{V}/\dot{Q}$ ratio and the venous partial pressures of O_2 and CO_2. With increasing exercise intensity, venous PO_2 goes down and venous PCO_2 goes up. These changes would be expected to decrease P_AO_2 and increase P_ACO_2. The only thing that can save the day is an increase in the $\dot{V}/\dot{Q}$ ratio. And that is exactly what happens. The $\dot{V}/\dot{Q}$ ratio increases in proportion to the intensity of exercise. Ventilation increases just enough in relation to the increase in cardiac output to keep the composition of alveolar air constant.

Question:
What accounts for the hyperpnea of exercise? Arterial chemoreceptors have been ruled out and no one has ever been able to find venous chemoreceptors. So what about pulmonary alveolar receptors? We already know there are alveolar O_2 receptors that are involved in hypoxic vasoconstriction. But are there alveolar O_2 or CO_2 receptors that send information to the medulla to regulate breathing and keep the composition of alveolar air constant?

Chapter 15

Altitude and Depth

Part 1: High Altitude

Topic 1: Atmospheric Pressure and Altitude

Figure 1
Atmospheric pressure decreases exponentially with altitude as shown in Figure 1. Pressure halves with each 18,000 ft of altitude.

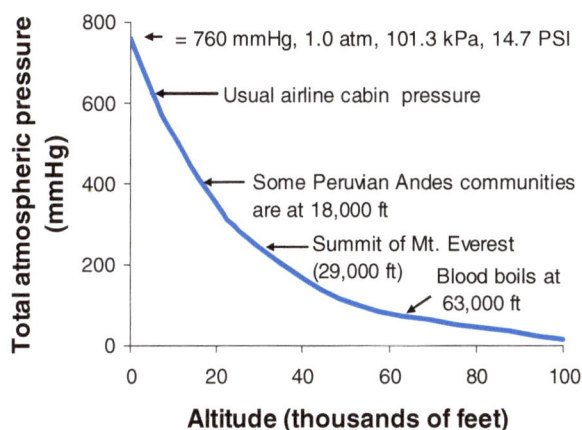

Figure 1. Atmospheric pressure as a function of altitude.

The concentration of oxygen remains the same at all altitudes (21% in dry air). Therefore, the partial pressure of oxygen decreases with altitude in proportion to the exponential decrease in total pressure. Coping with this drop in ambient PO_2 is crucially important in aviation, ballooning, and mountain climbing.

Topic 2: Atmospheric PO_2 and Alveolar PO_2 with Increasing Altitude

Figure 2
In ambient air and also in the alveoli, PO_2 decreases exponentially with altitude. For this figure, alveolar PO_2 is calculated by the alveolar air equation (Chapter 4, Equation 9), assuming for the uncompensated curve a constant alveolar PCO_2 of 40 mmHg and a respiratory exchange ratio of 0.8.

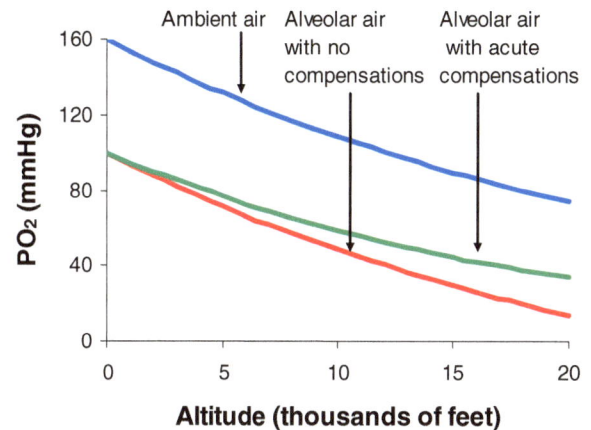

Figure 2. Ambient and alveolar PO_2 at increasing altitudes. Acute compensation takes place by increased ventilation and increased cardiac output.

Topic 3: Immediate Ventilatory Compensation

Figure 2 again
Ventilation increases with altitude, especially above about 5,000 ft. This effect is caused by hypoxic stimulation of arterial chemoreceptors (see Chapter 11).

The green curve in Figure 2 showing acute compensation is only approximate; its location depends on many factors including variations among individuals. The point is that increased alveolar ventilation is significantly increased and this increases P_AO_2 at all altitudes, becoming especially obvious above about 5,000 ft.

There is an additional minor factor. The trachealis muscle contracts. This muscle connects the ends of the tracheo-bronchial cartilages. Contraction results in a decreased diameter of the trachea and large bronchi, reducing anatomical dead space and, thereby, increasing alveolar ventilation. However, this good effect may be offset due to increased resistance to airflow through the bronchi.

Consequences of Increased Alveolar Ventilation

As ventilation increases with altitude, more carbon dioxide is blown off. Arterial and alveolar PCO_2 decrease and respiratory alkalosis develops. The decrease in $PaCO_2$ causes an alkalosis in the chemosensitive areas of the medulla; this tends to reduce ventilation (see Chapter 11). There is a fight between arterial chemoreceptors (trying to increase ventilation) and central chemoreceptors (trying to reduce it). As a result, alveolar ventilation only doubles or so. There is, however, a favorable effect of decreased alveolar PCO_2. This allows alveolar PO_2 to increase somewhat (see alveolar air equation).

One of the long term adaptations (acclimatization, see below) is that the central chemoreceptors gradually lose much of their responsiveness to low PCO_2. This allows for a much greater ventilatory response to hypoxemia and alveolar ventilation can eventually increase 4 or 5 fold.

Topic 4: Immediate Cardiac Output Compensation

You may recall that when the arterial chemoreceptors are stimulated by hypoxemia, they not only signal for increased pulmonary ventilation but also result in increased sympathetic activity to the heart. Therefore, cardiac output increases with increasing altitude.

Topic 5: Oxygen Delivery   Figure 3

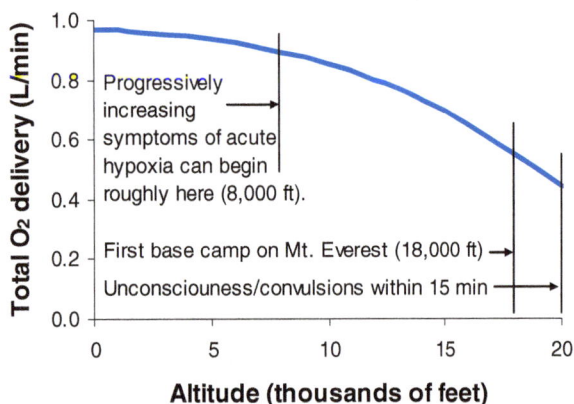

Figure 3. Total oxygen delivery with increasing altitude. O_2 delivery data shown here assumes acute compensations (increased ventilation and cardiac output) have taken place.

The most important thing is oxygen delivery to the metabolizing tissues. Total oxygen delivery is simply the oxygen content of arterial blood multiplied by cardiac output. Calculated total oxygen delivery at increasing altitude is shown in Figure 3.

Topic 6: Acute Mountain Sickness

People who ascend to roughly 8,000 feet or more, especially if they do so rapidly and stay there a day or so, sometimes develop uncomfortable and even dangerous symptoms. Early symptoms include the following:

- Headache
- Insomnia
- Dizziness or light-headedness
- Fatigue
- Loss of appetite
- Nausea/vomiting
- Tachycardia
- Dyspnea with mild exertion
- Drowsiness

Many of these symptoms can actually begin as low as 6,500 ft but may often be unnoticed or ignored.

More severe symptoms (usually seen at higher altitudes and/or longer exposures) include the following:

- Cyanosis
- Tightness in the chest
- Confusion
- Cough
- Decreased cognition
- Awkward gait
- Malaise
- Peripheral edema

Even more severe symptoms that may be life-threatening are:

- Pulmonary edema with dyspnea at rest
- Cerebral edema with gradual loss of consciousness

Pulmonary hypertension may also occur and is due to the increased cardiac output together with hypoxic vasoconstriction of pulmonary arterioles. It is thought that pulmonary hypertension is what leads to pulmonary edema, but the mechanism is not clear.

A person at altitude who is suffering from a subset of the above symptoms is said to have <u>acute mountain sickness</u>. The symptoms are caused by hypoxemia, hypocapnia (decreased $PaCO_2$), and alkalosis. Many of the CNS symptoms are probably caused mainly by cerebral <u>vasoconstriction</u> resulting from brain hypocapnia. Curiously, however, with longer exposure and/or higher altitudes cerebral <u>vasodilation</u> due to hypoxia may actually cause increased capillary blood pressure with resulting cerebral edema.

Treatment of Acute Mountain Sickness

The main thing is to get the patient to a lower altitude if that is possible. In the meantime, supplemental oxygen should be administered if that is possible.

Topic 7: Acclimatization

Over periods of days/weeks compensations occur that partially correct the problems with oxygen delivery and alkalosis, as long as the altitude is not too high. These adaptations are called acclimatization.

Renal Compensation for Respiratory Alkalosis

Renal elimination of bicarbonate and retention of H^+ brings blood pH back down toward normal. This happens over a period of a few days (see Chapter 12).

Cerebral Compensation for Cerebral Alkalosis

The bicarbonate concentration in cerebral spinal fluid gradually decreases, bringing CSF pH back down toward normal. Presumably this happens because a bicarbonate pump in the blood-brain barrier is activated and transports bicarbonate from CSF to capillary blood. It is also possible that a bicarbonate transporter in the choroid plexus (which secretes CSF) is inhibited.

Further Increase in Alveolar Ventilation

The brake on the increase in ventilation that is caused by central chemoreceptors is eased and there can be a far larger increase in ventilation – up to 4 or 5 fold, instead of the measly doubling before acclimatization.

Increased Hematocrit and Hemoglobin

When the kidneys sense hypoxemia they secrete erythropoietin. This hormone stimulates bone marrow to make red blood cells. The hematocrit can rise to 60% or so, and the hemoglobin concentration in blood can reach over 20 mg/dl (normal at sea level is about 15 mg/dl). As a result, the oxygen carrying capacity of blood goes up enormously. So does the viscosity of blood and this can raise peripheral resistance enough to be detrimental. In some cases this can actually be a maladaptation.

Increased 2,3-DPG in Red Cells

Recall that increased 2,3-diphosphoglycerate in red cells increases the P_{50} for oxygen binding to hemoglobin, *i.e.* reduces affinity (Chapter 7). At high altitude, the DPG concentration in red cells increases. The result is more complete oxygen release from Hb in the tissues. So not only is oxygen delivery to the tissues improved, but oxygen extraction from blood is also improved.

Increased Capillarity in Tissues

In many tissues, most notably the heart, increased capillarization is stimulated by hypoxemia. This further increases oxygen extraction.

Increased Oxidative Enzymes in Mitochondria

Over time at altitude, mitochondria develop a greater potential for oxidative metabolism due to more content of the enzymes involved in oxidative phosphorylation. This increases oxygen extraction even further.

Some of the above adaptations, including DPG, erythropoiesis, and angiogenesis, are mediated by an intracellular transcription factor called hypoxia-inducible factor 1 (HIF-1).

Topic 8: Chronic Mountain Sickness

Occasionally, someone who has been living at high altitude for a long time (say a year or longer) and is apparently well acclimatized, develops various symptoms such as headache, insomnia, cough, dyspnea, tachycardia, rales, liver enlargement, and peripheral edema. Hypoxemia is present, often with cyanosis. The patient always has pulmonary hypertension and usually severe polycythemia. The right ventricle is enlarged. The patient is diagnosed with right heart failure consequent to pulmonary hypertension and has what is called chronic mountain sickness (or Monge's disease). It is also known as <u>pulmonary hypertension-related high altitude heart disease</u>.

The cause of the pulmonary hypertension is increased cardiac output in the face of increased pulmonary vascular resistance. The latter is due to the combination of pulmonary hypoxic

vasoconstriction and increased blood viscosity caused by polycythemia. Thus, in this case polycythemia is a maladaptation.

Chronic mountain sickness can be fatal, but usually the patient recovers after being transported to lower altitude.

Part 2: Underwater Diving

Topic 1: Hydrostatic Pressure and Depth

Figure 4
As opposed to the <u>exponential</u> decline in atmospheric pressure with increasing altitude, the hydrostatic pressure in water increases <u>linearly</u> with depth. This difference is because air is compressible and water is not. At a depth of 33 ft, the pressure is twice atmospheric (at sea level) and increases another 760 mmHg with each additional 33 ft.

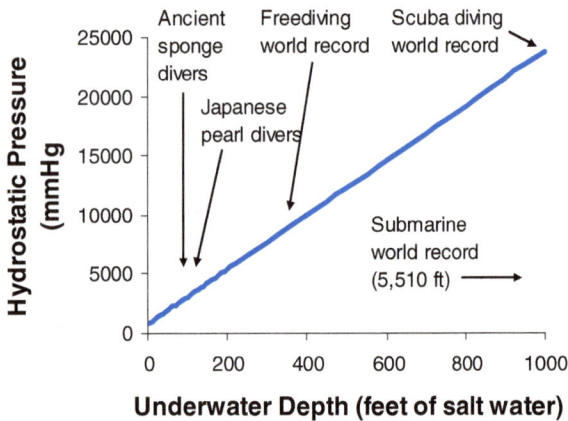

Figure 4. Linear increase in hydrostatic pressure with depth.

Topic 2: Shallow Immersion

Solid parts of the body are not compressible, but anything that is filled with air, such as the lungs, is compressible. At just a few feet under water, total lung capacity is not importantly changed, but FRC is markedly reduced because the increased pressure on the chest wall effectively adds to its normal elastic recoil force. The decrease in FRC decreases expiratory reserve volume while increasing inspiratory reserve volume. The work of inspiration

is considerably increased because of this excess in effective elastic recoil of the chest wall.

Increased pressure on the body surface decreases venous blood volume, increases central venous pressure, and consequently increases cardiac output. On the other hand increased body surface pressure squeezes down on resistance vessels, thereby increasing total peripheral resistance and reducing cardiac output. The overall effect on cardiac output is minor, at least in shallow water.

Can a person stay immersed while breathing through a long snorkel tube? Not over about 3 feet. This limitation is not as much of a dead space problem as it is a pressure problem; in fact it occurs even if the snorkel is fitted with a valve that makes expiration go directly into the water. The problem is that maximum inspiratory pressures cannot exceed roughly 75 mmHg. Consequently, when the water pressure is above this value (at about 3.3 ft) inspiration is impossible.

Topic 3: Freediving

Freediving is also called breath-hold diving. As hydrostatic pressure on the body surface increases, the lungs are compressed, and total pressure in the lungs becomes about equal to the hydrostatic pressure at any depth. At 33 ft, for example, total lung capacity is reduced by almost half (not quite, since the chest wall offers some resistance to compression) and intrapulmonary pressure nearly doubles. As total pressure in the lungs increases, so do all partial pressures.

As depth increases, P_AO_2 increases and this can be beneficial. However, P_ACO_2 also increases, thereby reducing the rate of diffusion from blood to alveoli leading to CO_2 retention. In fact P_ACO_2 can become greater than it is in blood with reversal of the direction of net diffusion. CO_2 retention can be a great problem in breath-hold diving partly because of its effect on the central chemoreceptors, which results in a powerful drive to breathe.

The human freediving world record for depth shown in Figure 4 is incredible (about 360 ft), but an ordinary whale can beat this by far, descending to more than 2500 ft and staying there for more than an hour.

Topic 4: Scuba Diving

There have been a number of devices that allow for breathing while deep under water, for example the diving bell, the underwater caisson, the diving helmet, scuba gear, and submarines. We will focus on scuba diving but much of the information is applicable to the other devices.

Scuba means self-contained underwater breathing apparatus. It was developed most notably by Jacques Cousteau in 1943. In scuba diving, the gas mixture is inhaled from a tank that goes along with the diver, and the breathing apparatus keeps the gas at ambient pressure. Therefore, intrapulmonary pressure nearly equals body surface pressure and the problem with inhaling against a high pressure is obviated. However, a different problem results from the fact that as the pressure of inspired gas increases, so does its density. The turbulent flow in the upper airways is very sensitive to air density. As density increases, resistance to flow increases and the work of breathing goes up. Replacing nitrogen with helium in the gas mixture reduces this problem since the density of helium is much less than that of nitrogen. In addition, the viscosity of helium is greater than that of nitrogen. Decreased density and increased viscosity both decrease the likelihood of turbulent flow rather than laminar flow in smaller airways as can be seen by examining the equation for Reynolds number (Chapter 3, p. 28). Since turbulent flow requires a much greater driving force for a given flow rate, replacing nitrogen with helium significantly reduces the work of breathing.

Poisonous Effects of Compressed Gases

Nitrogen Narcosis

After an hour or so at roughly 150 ft or more, divers breathing compressed air can get nitrogen narcosis. Symptoms include giddiness and a euphoric feeling that is sometimes called *rapture of the deep*. At greater depths and times, weakness, drowsiness,

clumsiness, and even coma can set in and the diver becomes useless and in danger.

The cause of nitrogen narcosis is not well understood, but N_2 at high partial pressure dissolves appreciably in lipids, including neuronal cell membranes in the brain. High lipid solubility is a common property of gaseous general anesthetics. Helium is much less soluble in lipids than is nitrogen, and replacing nitrogen with helium in the gas mixture pretty much solves the problem.

Oxygen Toxicity

At high partial pressure, oxygen can be toxic due to generation of oxygen free radicals such as peroxide, and superoxide at a rate that exceeds the ability of free radical scavengers (*e.g.* peroxidase, catalase, and superoxide dismutase) to remove them. If 100% oxygen is breathed for an hour or so, even at 1 atm, the pulmonary epithelium can be damaged, resulting in pulmonary congestion, pulmonary edema, and atelectasis. At high ambient pressures as in scuba diving, a more general problem may appear that especially involves the brain. Symptoms can include twitching, dizziness, irritability, and eventually disorientation, seizures, and coma. So divers beware.

The solution to the problem is to replace some of the oxygen in the gas mixture with helium.

Decompression Sickness

At depth, N_2 dissolves in body water and especially in body fats. Upon decompression N_2 diffuses out of body water and fat, and can form tiny bubbles. If ascent is too rapid, larger bubbles can form and can cause trouble. Small N_2 bubbles in venous blood are mostly filtered out in the lungs and don't usually cause problems. Rarely, however, N_2 bubbles can cause pulmonary symptoms such as substernal pain, cough, dyspnea, and pulmonary hypertension, and the person is said to have the chokes. Even more rarely, bubbles can get through the lungs and form arterial emboli that can block cerebral blood flow with consequent stroke. Sometimes N_2 bubbles that form in joints cause severe pain known as the bends.

The treatment for decompression sickness is recompression. Prevention is by using helium in the gas mixture, and by slow ascent, often according to one of several decompression schedules.

Hurray for Helium!

Helium helps. It is not nearly as soluble in water and fat as is nitrogen. Therefore, not nearly as much comes out of solution upon decompression and bubbles are not as likely to form.

Part 3: What Can Go Wrong?

All sorts of mechanical and judgment things can go wrong at altitude and depth, but we will limit this list to respiratory pathophysiology and medicine. Most of these problems have been discussed above.

Altitude

Hypoxemia, hypocapnia, and alkalosis
Acute mountain sickness
Chronic mountain sickness

Depth

Nitrogen narcosis
Oxygen toxicity
Decompression sickness

Chapter 16

Birth and Aging

Part 1: Birth

Topic 1: Fetal Arrangement of the Cardiovascular and Pulmonary Systems

Figure 1

The fetal circulation has certain structures that are not normally functional in adults. These are the foramen ovale, the ductus arteriosus, the ductus venosus and, of course, the two umbilical arteries and the umbilical vein. These structures are colored red in Figure 1.

The fetus, of course, cannot breathe air. All respiratory gas exchange takes place across the placenta. The placenta in not a good gas exchanger compared to postnatal lungs. Blood enters the placenta in the umbilical arteries with a PO_2 of about 23 mmHg, and leaves in the umbilical vein with a PO_2 of about 30 mmHg. This is far from the degree of equilibration accomplished in postnatal lungs.

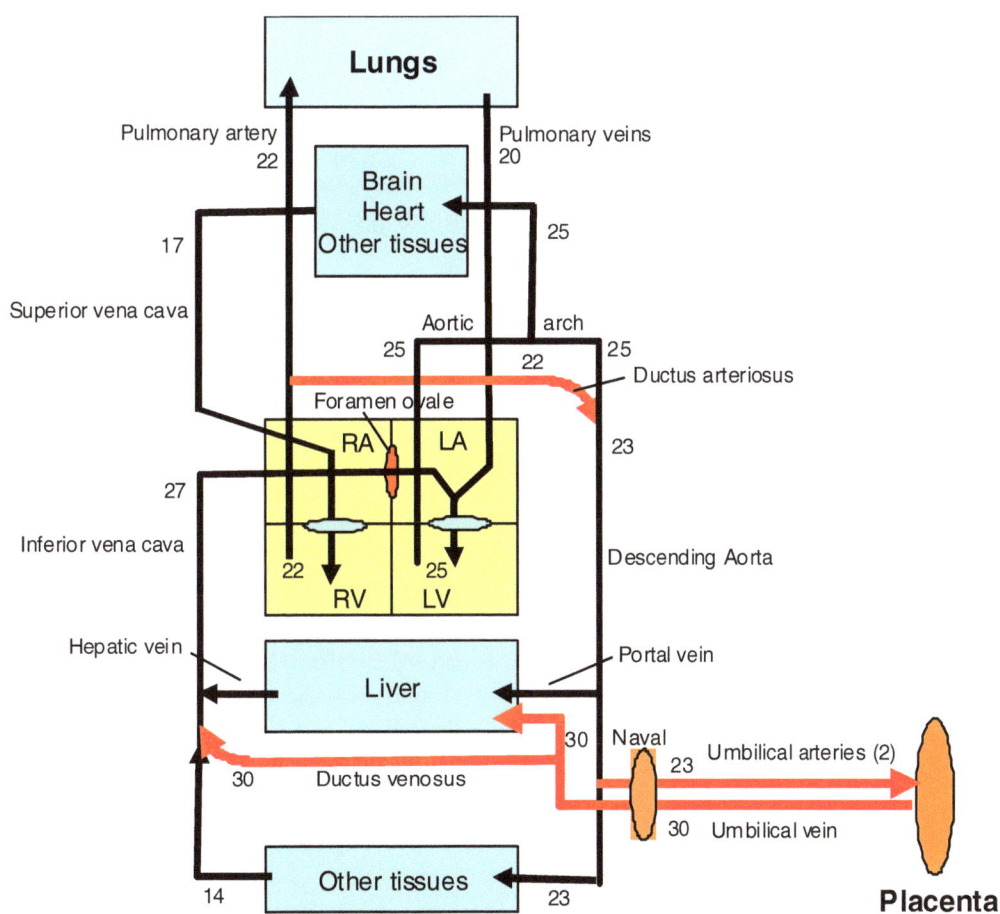

Figure 1. Diagram of the fetal circulation. Permanent blood vessels are black. The red structures are temporary. They normally do not function after birth. They accomplish fetal blood flow through the placenta and diversion of blood flow away from the lungs. See text for description. The numbers are for approximate PO_2 in mmHg.

The umbilical vein sends one branch to the liver and another directly to the inferior vena cava, bypassing the liver. Each of these branches carries about ½ the total flow. The branch to the inferior vena cava is called the <u>ductus venosus</u>. Umbilical venous blood is joined in the inferior vena cava by blood from the liver and other tissues, and eventually reaches the right atrium. Most of this blood flows preferential into the left atrium (rather than the right ventricle) through the <u>foramen ovale</u>. This flow is apparently directed by the blood momentum vector which points toward the foramen ovale and there is incomplete mixing with blood from the superior vena cava. Moreover, blood from the placenta is not well mixed in the vena cava with venous blood from other organs and this separation of flows is partially maintained in the right atrium. Most of the relatively deoxygenated blood from metabolizing tissues flows into the right ventricle. The result is that blood entering the left atrium through the foramen ovale is not diluted extensively by venous blood from other tissues. Left atrial blood enters the left ventricle through the mitral valve and is then pumped into the aorta with a PO_2 of about 25 mmHg. This PO_2 is somewhat higher than it is in the descending aorta. Thus the brain and heart get maximally oxygenated blood. This is good.

Blood entering the right atrium from the superior vena cava has a PO_2 of roughly 17 mmHg. It flows somewhat preferentially through the tricuspid valve into the right ventricle. The right ventricle pumps blood into the pulmonary artery where the PO_2 is about 22 mmHg, having been elevated by some mixing with inferior vena caval blood in the right atrium.

Most of the blood that enters the pulmonary artery never reaches the lungs; about 90% of it flows through the <u>ductus arteriosus</u> into the aorta. This blood mixes with blood pumped from the left ventricle and its PO_2 is raised to about 23 mmHg. The output of the left ventricle is only about half that of the right ventricle. Therefore, most of the blood in the descending aorta gets there *via* the ductus arteriosus rather than the left ventricle.

Why does most of the blood pumped by the right ventricle flow through the ductus arteriosus to the aorta rather than through the lungs to the pulmonary veins? The answer is that pulmonary vascular resistance in the fetus is very high, about 10 times higher than systemic vascular resistance. This

situation is advantageous for the fetus since gas exchange occurs in the placenta rather than the lungs.

Topic 2: Changes at Birth

Spectacular and profound changes occur at birth. During the birthing process the umbilical arteries close. This event occurs even if the umbilicus is not promptly tied and cut. It is not really understood what causes this. The umbilical arteries have thick walls that are very muscular, and are quite responsive to a variety of humoral agents including epinephrine, norepinephrine, angiotensin II, and O_2, but what is actually responsible for their timely constriction seems not to be known. Shutdown of the umbilical circulation greatly increases systemic vascular resistance in the infant, and this increases aortic pressure and left atrial pressure. Closure of the umbilical artery also decreases pressure in the inferior vena cava and right atrium. Elevated pressure in the left atrium, together with reduced pressure in the right atrium, causes the flap-like valve covering the left side of the foramen ovale to shut. Now all blood flowing into the right atrium goes into the right ventricle and is pumped into the pulmonary artery.

Immediately after shutdown of the umbilical circulation, arterial PO_2 decreases and arterial PCO_2 increases. Apparently at this same moment the sensitivity of arterial chemoreceptors increases. The inspiratory regions in the medulla oblongata are activated by the chemoreceptors and the infant takes its first breath of air. The lungs had been filled during most of fetal life to about 40% of total lung capacity (TLC) with liquid secreted by alveolar epithelium. This volume roughly equals the eventual functional residual capacity (FRC). Shortly before birth, however, this fluid secretion stops and a large fraction of lung liquid is actively absorbed into the blood and a little into lymph. Additional liquid is squeezed out of the lungs during the birthing process. Thus, in the late stages of birth the lungs contain little liquid.

Expansion of the lungs during the first breath is very difficult because as the alveoli start to fill with air the developing air-liquid interface provides a lot of surface tension. Intrapleural pressure must be greatly reduced (to roughly minus 60 mmHg) by action of the surprisingly strong muscles of inspiration. These muscles have been trained to some degree by little gasps that take place during fetal life. These gasps start near the end of the first trimester, but they greatly diminish shortly before birth. The presence of pulmonary surfactant, secreted by type II epithelial cells fairly late in fetal life, greatly reduces alveolar surface tension and facilitates inspiration. The first expiration leaves some air in the lungs and subsequent breaths quickly result in a steady amount of end-tidal volume, the FRC. Following the first breath, subsequent inspirations gradually become much easier due partly to clearance of liquid in airways and perhaps more effective distribution of surfactant.

In the meantime, pulmonary vascular resistance drops to about 10% of its fetal value. This, together with the increase in systemic vascular resistance, the rise in left atrial pressure, and the fall in right atrial pressure cause pulmonary venous blood to flow mainly through the lungs instead of through the ductus arteriosus. In fact, the direction of blood flow through the ductus arteriosus actually reverses. The ductus arteriosus then constricts, probably as a result of better oxygenation. Now, all the blood pumped by the right ventricle into the pulmonary artery continues on through the lungs. This happens at essentially the same time that the lungs have filled with air and are ready to replace the placenta as the respiratory gas exchanger.

There are at least two reasons for the sudden drop in pulmonary vascular resistance at birth:

- Expansion of the lungs with the first breath not only expands the alveoli, but also the pulmonary blood vessels, including the arterioles.
- Increased PO_2 in the alveoli reverses the hypoxic vasoconstriction that had previously been keeping the arterioles constricted.

Topic 3: Postnatal Changes

Now the baby has a cardio-pulmonary system that functions in the adult manner. Venous blood from all tissues flows to the right heart, is pumped through the lungs, and flows on to the left heart, which pumps arterialized blood to all tissues. But there is still some mopping up to be done.

Umbilical Vessels and Ductus Venosus
The umbilical arteries and vein and the ductus venosus, now with no blood flow, no nutrition, and no oxygenation, shrivel up and disappear. This happens after birth over a period of several hours to days. Blood flow to the liver becomes entirely from the portal vein and hepatic artery.

Ductus Arteriosus
As aortic pressure increases, and pulmonary artery pressure decreases, the direction of flow through the ductus arteriosus reverses, so that well-oxygenated blood flows through it. The increase in PO_2 causes the ductus arteriosus to constrict and flow is reduced to zero within a few hours or days (or sometimes longer). Even after complete obstruction, with no O_2 supply, the ductus arteriosus remains closed. This may be due to a decline in prostacyclin at birth, which had been causing active smooth muscle relaxation. The non-functional ductus arteriosus eventually disappears. Rarely, the ductus arteriosus remains partly open causing a left-to-right shunt. This problem can be corrected surgically.

Foramen Ovale
The closed valve flap gradually seals to the interatrial septum. Complete sealing can take a few days or even months, in fact in about 15% to 20% of people sealing is never complete. Even in these people, right to left shunting does not occur because the pressure difference is in the wrong direction, and left to right shunting is not often a problem because the valve flap, though not completely sealed, still works as a one-way valve. Rarely, a small embolus from a deep venous thrombosis can get through a partially patent foramen ovale and cause a stroke.

Thickness of Ventricular Walls
In the fetus, right and left ventricular wall thicknesses are about the same. At birth, pulmonary artery pressure drops because of the decrease in pulmonary vascular resistance. Consequently, afterload to the right ventricle drastically decreases and, over a few weeks, its muscle atrophies until its wall thickness is much less than that of the left ventricle, which has hypertrophied over this same time period due to the rise in left ventricular afterload.

Part 2: Aging

Certain pulmonary functions go downhill with age. This happens even in normal people and non-smokers. Some of these changes start as early as 20 years of age.

Topic 1: Lungs

Connective tissue fibers in the parenchyma of the lungs degenerate with age, much as in emphysema but far less severe. This has the following consequences:

Increased Compliance
Degeneration of connective tissue leads to increased lung compliance and decreased tendency of the lungs to recoil.

Decreased Numbers of Alveoli
Degeneration of connective tissue also leads to confluence of alveoli with decreased alveolar surface area. In addition, alveolar capillarity decreases. Therefore, diffusion capacity measured by the carbon monoxide technique ($D_L CO$, see Chapter 6, p. 60) gradually declines with age.

Airway Collapse
Loss of radial traction due to connective tissue degeneration causes small airways to become somewhat skinnier with a slight increase in airway resistance. More importantly, dynamic airway collapse occurs at progressively higher lung volumes, which leads to greater functional residual capacity.

$\dot{V}/\dot{Q}$ Mismatch and A-a PO_2 Difference
Collapse of small airways leads to hypoventilated alveoli. The resulting decrease in the $\dot{V}/\dot{Q}$ ratio causes a decrease in arterial PO_2 and an increase in the A-a PO_2 difference. A common rule of thumb (Chapter 10, p. 87) is that the A-a PO_2 difference (in mmHg) should not be greater than about Age/4 + 4.

Decreased $D_L CO$ may contribute slightly to this effect, but it is mostly due to $\dot{V}/\dot{Q}$ mismatch.

Topic 2: Chest Wall

With aging, the chest wall becomes stiffer and its compliance decreases. During inspiration from FRC, the chest wall tries to recoil more forcefully. But during forceful expiration from FRC, the chest wall tries to expand more forcefully. These changes increase the work of breathing.

Topic 3: Muscles

The muscles of respiration become weaker with aging. Also the frequency of motor neuron firing to the muscles of inspiration diminishes.

Topic 4: Lung Volumes   Figure 2

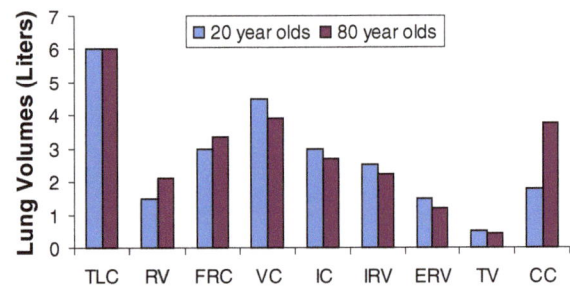

Figure 2. Changes in standard lung volumes with aging – 20 years *vs.* 80 years. The data are for a healthy person having a total lung capacity of 6.0 liters at age 20. We assume that this person remains well, has never been a smoker, and has not been exposed chronically to environmental or industrial toxins and irritants. TLC = total lung capacity, RV = residual volume, FRC = functional residual capacity, VC = vital capacity, IC = inspiratory capacity, IRV = inspiratory reserve volume, ERV = expiratory reserve volume, TV = tidal volume, CC = closing capacity. Closing capacity is the lung volume during expiration at which the small airways begin the process of dynamic airway collapse (see Chapter 3, p. 24). Most of the above data were gleaned from a chart in Levitsky's *Pulmonary Physiology, 6th Ed.*, p. 82, and are only approximate.

Consider the following effects of aging on lung volumes:

- TLC remains fairly constant.
- RV increases substantially. This is mainly due to the drop in elastic recoil of the lungs. Decreased strength of expiratory muscles also contributes.

- FRC increases because of the increase in RV.
- VC decreases because of the increase in RV together with the fact that TLC remains constant.
- IC decreases due to the increase in FRC.
- IRV decreases due to the increase in FRC.
- ERV decreases due to the fact that RV increases relatively more that does FRC.
- TV decreases a little because the muscles of inspiration get weaker, especially the diaphragm.
- CC (closing capacity, see Figure 2 legend) increases a lot. Roughly it doubles. This is because the phenomenon of dynamic airway collapse begins earlier during expiration, *i.e.* at greater lung volume. The cause is degeneration of lung parenchymal connective tissue fibers with reduced radial traction on small airways. Figure 2 shows that CC may actually rise slightly above FRC. When this happens, passive expiration to FRC may encounter some degree of dynamic airway collapse with a consequent increase in airway resistance leading possibly to dyspnea even at rest.

Most of these changes with aging are minimal, except for the substantial increase in RV and for the extreme increase in CC.

Topic 5: Pulmonary Function Tests

Forced one second expiration (FEV_1) declines with age, but so does forced vital capacity (FVC). The ratio FEV_1/FVC remains essentially unchanged. See Appendix 1 for description and interpretation of these tests.

Topic 6: Reflexes

The pulmonary responses to arterial PO_2 and PCO_2 diminish with age. This is apparently because the peripheral and central chemoreceptors become less sensitive.

Topic 7: Maximum Exercise Capacity

Maximum exercise capacity and $\dot{V}O_2$ max both decline with age. This is mainly due to loss of muscle mass, especially at advanced age and especially in sedentary people. This decline is also partly due to the decrease, during aging, in the ability to raise heart rate. The approximate rule of thumb for maximum heart rate during exercise is:

$$Max\ HR = 220 - Age$$

Topic 8: Defense Mechanisms

The effectiveness of the mucociliary escalator declines with age. This may contribute to the fact that many old people (even non-smokers) cough quite a bit each morning. There are also declines in immune responses and probably in the cough reflex.

Topic 9: Diseases

Progressive pulmonary diseases by definition get worse with age. These include obstructive and restrictive pulmonary diseases. In addition, susceptibility to various pulmonary diseases increases with aging.

Topic 10: Outcomes

In spite of all the above effects of aging on pulmonary functions, few if any noticeable symptoms occur at rest in healthy, non-smoking old people who have not been exposed chronically to environmental toxins and irritants. However, during exercise old people are more susceptible to dyspnea due especially to the increase in CC.

Appendix 1

Pulmonary Function Tests

Pulmonary function testing (PFT) is done for aiding diagnosis, assessing severity, and for following disease progression and treatment effectiveness.

Topic 1: Lung Volumes

Figure 1

This figure shows that in obstructive pulmonary diseases nearly all of the standard lung volumes are increased (hyperinflation), and in restrictive pulmonary diseases nearly all are decreased (hypoinflation). Many of these volumes require only simple spirometry. The first three (TLC, RV and FRC) also need a separate measurement of residual volume, preferably with body plethysmography. Vital capacity (VC) and inspiratory capacity (IC) are the simplest measures to distinguish between an obstructive problem and a restrictive problem using nothing but simple spirometry.

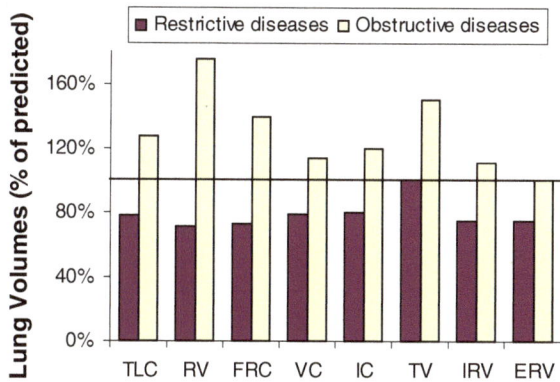

Figure 1. Relative lung volumes in obstructive and restrictive diseases. Data are expressed as percentages of predicted, which means normal corrected for size, age, and gender. Data above the horizontal line are consistent with hyperinflation and data below the horizontal line are consistent with hypoinflation. The data used for constructing this chart are from C.L. Scanlon *et al.*, *Egan's Fundamentals of Respiratory Care, 6th Ed.*, 1995.

It should be understood that the actual values shown in Figure 1 are very approximate and really just illustrate trends – up or down. They do not take account of variations among each particular disease and its severity.

Topic 2: Forced Expiration

A very important procedure using a modern spirometer (Chapter 2, p. 8) is the forced expiration maneuver following a full inspiration. The subject is instructed (and strongly encouraged) to breathe out as fast as possible. Two different relationships can be recorded: volume exhaled as a function of time, and rate of exhalation as a function of lung volume.

Volume Out *vs.* Time
Figure2
This figure shows the decline in total lung volume during 1) a forced expiration for a normal person, 2) someone having an obstructive disorder, and 3) someone with a restrictive disorder. The subjects are presumed matched for size, age, and gender.

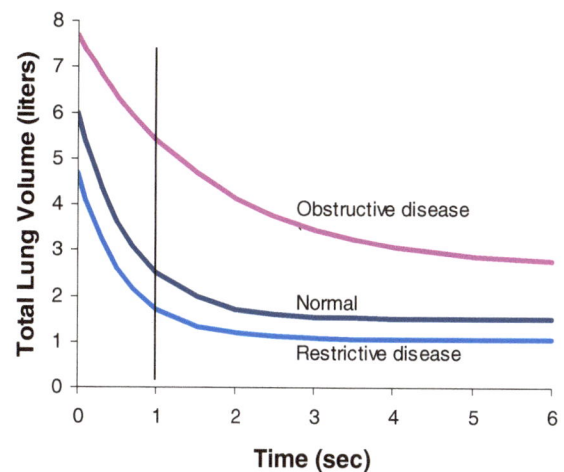

Figure 2. Forced expiration following a full inspiration. Lung volume is plotted against time during the forced expiration. A vertical line is drawn at 1.0 sec since the volume forcefully exhaled by 1.0 sec is often used for assessing the ease of exhalation.

Obviously the upper curve shows hyperinflation with difficulty in forcefully exhaling; the diagnosis of obstructive disease is indicated. The lower curve shows some hypoinflation with no apparent difficulty in exhaling; restrictive disease might be suspected. For quantitation, the volume exhaled within 1.0 sec is measured. This is called the forced expiratory volume$_1$ (FEV$_1$). It is especially useful to divide FEV$_1$ by the forced vital capacity, FVC, to obtain a value called FEV$_1$/FVC, or just FEV%. The value of FEV% is considerably decreased in obstructive disease and either not changed or increased a little in restrictive disease. The relevant calculated values for the data shown in Figure 2 are listed in Table 1.

Table 1

	Normal	Obstructive	Restrictive
FVC	4.5 L	5.04 L	3.61 L
FEV$_1$	3.5 L	2.28 L	2.95 L
FEV$_1$/FVC	78 %	45.2 %	81.7 %

Rate Out *vs.* Lung Volume
Figure 3

The flow rate (usually in liters/sec) at any lung volume is the slope of the volume *vs.* time relationship and can be calculated electronically by the instrument. In Figure 3, flow rate is plotted against lung volume as it changes from TLC to RV during the forced expiration.

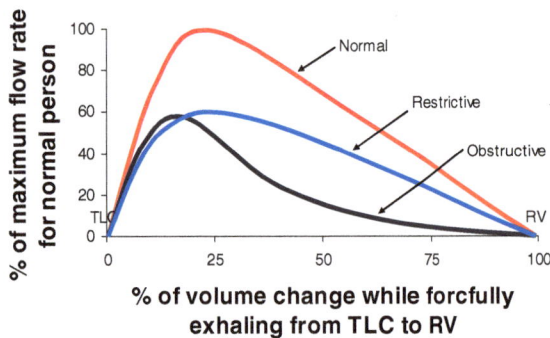

Figure 3. Forced expiratory flow-volume curves, showing qualitatively the effects of obstructive and restrictive pulmonary diseases. Understand that while all three curves eventually reach 100%, this is with respect to the VC for each particular condition. It takes much longer to reach RV in obstructive disease and less in restrictive than it does normally.

In obstructive disease, the curve becomes concave-up after 25% or so of the vital capacity has been exhaled. This curvature results from dynamic airway compression (Chapter 3), which starts much earlier than it normally does. The lower than normal flow rates in restrictive diseases do not result from obstruction but simply from the fact that the lung volumes are less.

It is especially useful to compare flow rates at certain prescribed degrees of forced expiration, often at 50% or 75%. Other indices are also used such as the peak expiratory flow rate (PEF or PEFR), average forced expiratory flow rate between 25% and 75% (FEF$_{25\%-75\%}$), forced expiratory time (FET), and slow vital capacity (SVC).

Upper airway obstruction can be distinguished from lower airway obstruction using flow-volume curves, but that takes us too far for this book.

Inspiratory flow-volume relationships can also be of value, but will not be discussed here.

Topic 3: Other Common Tests

Airway Resistance
Airway resistance, R$_{AW}$, can be measured using a body plethysmograph, which can determine alveolar pressure (P$_A$), airway opening pressure (P$_{AO}$), and flow rate simultaneously. The equation for airway resistance is:

$$R_{AW} = \frac{P_A - P_{AO}}{Flow\ rate}$$

Static Lung Compliance
Measurement of static lung compliance requires measuring the intrapleural pressure, for which an esophageal tube is used. The subject inspires to TLC and then passively exhales incrementally to FRC. After each increment, the intrapleural pressure is measured. The volume exhaled with each increment divided by the change in intrapleural pressure is the expiratory compliance.

Maximum Inspiratory and Expiratory Pressures
Again, an esophageal tube is required for measuring maximum inspiratory pressure (MIP) and maximum expiratory pressure (MEP). These are tests of respiratory muscle strength.

Diffusing Capacity
Measurement of lung diffusing capacity using carbon monoxide (D$_L$CO) was discussed in Chapter 6, p. 48-49.

Arterial Blood Gas Analysis

Arterial PO_2 and PCO_2 are determined from arterial blood samples using electrodes. Arterial pH is then calculated from the Henderson-Hasselbalch equation (Chapter 12). Alternatively, pH can be measured directly with a pH-sensitive glass electrode.

Arterial PCO_2 can be used in the alveolar gas equation (Chapter 4, p. 33) for estimating alveolar PO_2, which can then be compared to arterial PO_2 to get the A-a PO_2 difference.

Topic 4: A Diagnostic Chart

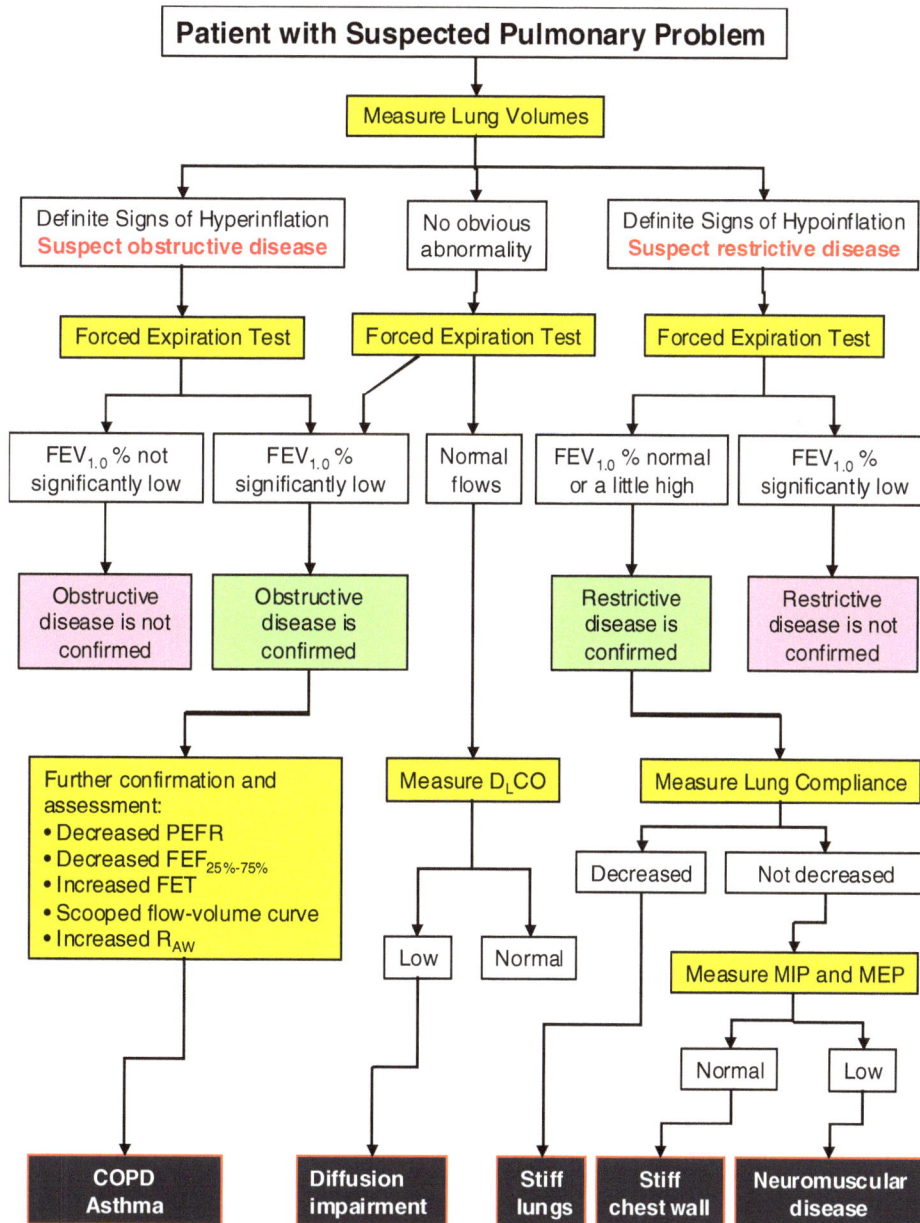

Patient with Suspected Pulmonary Problem

Measure Lung Volumes

| Definite Signs of Hyperinflation **Suspect obstructive disease** | No obvious abnormality | Definite Signs of Hypoinflation **Suspect restrictive disease** |

Forced Expiration Test — Forced Expiration Test — Forced Expiration Test

| $FEV_{1.0}$ % not significantly low | $FEV_{1.0}$ % significantly low | Normal flows | $FEV_{1.0}$ % normal or a little high | $FEV_{1.0}$ % significantly low |

| Obstructive disease is not confirmed | Obstructive disease is confirmed | Restrictive disease is confirmed | Restrictive disease is not confirmed |

Further confirmation and assessment:
• Decreased PEFR
• Decreased $FEF_{25\%-75\%}$
• Increased FET
• Scooped flow-volume curve
• Increased R_{AW}

Measure D_LCO

Measure Lung Compliance

| Decreased | Not decreased |

| Low | Normal |

Measure MIP and MEP

| Normal | Low |

COPD Asthma **Diffusion impairment** **Stiff lungs** **Stiff chest wall** **Neuromuscular disease**

Much of this chart is modified from M.K. Younes and J.E. Remmers, <u>Laboratory Evaluation of Respiratory Disease</u>, in *Continuing Education* <u>6</u> *(2)*, 1977. The yellow boxes designate the tests, the white boxes are the results, and the black boxes are the diagnoses.

Appendix 2

Equations

This appendix lists some important equations used in pulmonary physiology. Their order of appearance is the same as in the main text. Derivations are not given here.

Total Airway Resistance (p. 22)

$$R_{AW} = \frac{P_A - P_{AO}}{\dot{V}}$$

R_{AW} = airway resistance
P_A = alveolar pressure
P_{AO} = airway opening pressure (usually the same as atmospheric pressure)
$\dot{V}$ = rate of air flow

Reynolds Number (p. 23)
(Determines the likeliness of turbulent flow through a tube)

$$Re = \frac{\bar{v}\,\rho\,r}{\eta}$$

$\bar{v}$ = mean velocity of flow
ρ = density of fluid
r = tube radius
η = viscosity.
Re = Reynolds number

Resistance to Flow through a Tube (p. 23)
According to the Poiseuille equation, resistance through a straight, rigid, cylindrical, tube during laminar flow is given by:

$$R = \frac{8\,\eta\,l}{\pi\,r^4}$$

R = resistance
η = viscosity
l = length
r = radius

Bohr Equation (p. 30)

$$V_{Dp} = V_T\,\frac{P_{Af}CO_2 - P_E CO_2}{P_{Af}CO_2}$$

V_{Dp} = physiologic dead space
V_T = tidal volume
$P_{Af}CO_2$ = PCO_2 in functional alveolar air
$P_E CO_2$ = CO_2 in mixed expired air (expired dead space air mixed with expired alveolar air)

Alveolar Carbon Dioxide Equation (p.32)

$$F_A CO_2 = \frac{\dot{V}_E CO_2}{\dot{V}_A}$$

$F_A CO_2$ = fractional concentration of carbon dioxide in alveolar air (humidified)
$\dot{V}_E CO_2$ = volume of carbon dioxide exhaled in one minute (same as the amount produced by metabolism in one minute)
$\dot{V}_A$ = volume of alveolar air exhaled in one minute

Often the following form of this equation is used where the fractional concentration in alveolar air has been converted to partial pressure by multiplying by atmospheric pressure:

$$P_A CO_2 = \frac{\dot{V}_E CO_2}{\dot{V}_A} \times P_{atm}$$

$P_A CO_2$ = partial pressure of CO_2 in alveolar air
P_{atm} = atmospheric pressure

In making calculations, it is important to remember to express the rate of CO_2 elimination and the rate of alveolar ventilation in the same units (*e.g.* either ml/sec or liters/min)

The important thing to note from this equation is that alveolar CO_2, either fractional concentration or partial pressure, is inversely proportional to alveolar ventilation, assuming a constant rate of CO_2 production.

Since arterial PCO_2 is usually the same as alveolar PCO_2, the equation can also be written:

$$P_aCO_2 = \frac{\dot{V}_E CO_2}{\dot{V}_A} \times P_{atm}$$

Alveolar Oxygen Equation (p. 33)

$$F_AO_2 = F_IO_2 - \frac{\dot{V}O_2 consumed}{\dot{V}_A}$$

F_AO_2 = fractional concentration of oxygen in alveolar air

$\dot{V}_EO_2$ = volume of oxygen exhaled in one minute

$\dot{V}_A$ = volume of alveolar air exhaled in one minute

F_IO_2 = fractional concentration of oxygen in humidified inspired air

Alveolar Air Equation (p. 33)

$$P_AO_2 = P_IO_2 - \frac{P_ACO_2}{R} + \left\{ P_ACO_2 \times F_IO_2 \times \left(\frac{1}{R} - 1\right) \right\}$$

P_AO_2 = partial pressure of oxygen in alveolar air

P_IO_2 = partial pressure of oxygen in humidified inspired air

P_ACO_2 = partial pressure of carbon dioxide in alveolar air

F_IO_2 = fractional concentration of oxygen in <u>dry</u> inspired air (0.21)

R = respiratory exchange ratio

The entire term in brackets on the right amounts to only about 2 mmHg. Therefore, it is often ignored and the following simplified equation is used:

$$P_AO_2 = P_IO_2 - \frac{P_ACO_2}{R}$$

Pulmonary Vascular Resistance (p. 37)

$$PVR = \frac{mPAP - mPVP}{CO}$$

PVR = pulmonary vascular resistance
mPAP = mean pulmonary artery pressure
mPVP = mean pulmonary vein pressure
CO = cardiac output

Net Filtration Pressure (p. 42)

$$P_{net} = (P_c - P_i) - \sigma (\pi_c - \pi_i)$$

P_{net} = net filtration pressure
P_c = capillary hydrostatic pressure
P_i = interstitial hydrostatic pressure
π_c = capillary oncotic pressure (due to plasma proteins)
π_i = interstitial oncotic pressure (due to interstitial proteins and glycosaminoglycans)
σ = the reflection coefficient

Fick's Law for Rate of Gas Diffusion across a Membrane (p. 46)

$$Rate = A \cdot D_m \cdot s \cdot \frac{P_1 - P_2}{w}$$

A = area of the membrane
D_m = diffusion coefficient of the gas in the membrane
w = thickness of the membrane
s = solubility of the gas in the membrane
P_1 and P_2 are the partial pressures of the gas in the solutions bathing the two sides of the membrane

Shunt Equation (p. 66)

$$\frac{Q_S}{Q_T} = \frac{C_N O_2 - CaO_2}{C_N O_2 - CvO_2}$$

Q_T = total cardiac output
Q_S = rate of shunt flow
CaO_2 = O_2 concentration in aortic blood
CvO_2 = O_2 concentration in mixed venous blood
$C_N O_2$ = O_2 concentration in blood leaving normally ventilated alveoli

Henderson-Hasselbalch Equation (p. 87)

$$pH = 6.1 + \log \frac{[HCO_3^-]}{0.03 \times PaCO_2}$$

$$pH = \log \frac{1}{[H^+]}$$

$[HCO_3^-]$ = bicarbonate concentration
$PaCO_2$ = partial pressure of carbon dioxide

Symbols Commonly Used in Pulmonary Physiology and Medicine

Lung Volumes
Tidal	TV (V_T)
Dead space	V_D
Alveolar	V_A
Inspiratory reserve	IRV
Expiratory reserve	ERV
Residual	RV
Minimal	MV

Lung Capacities
Total	TLC
Vital	VC
Inspiratory	IC
Functional residual	FRC

Pressures
Barometric	P_B
Airway opening	P_{AO}
Body surface	P_{BS}
Alveolar	P_A
Intrapleural	P_{PL}
Maximum inspiratory	MIP
Maximum expiratory	MEP
Equal pressure point	EPP

Pressure Differences
Transairway	P_{TA}
Transpulmonary	P_{TP}
Translung	P_L
Transthoracic	P_W
Transrespiratory	P_{RS}

Partial Pressures
Arterial O_2	PaO_2
Arterial CO_2	$PaCO_2$
Alveolar O_2	P_AO_2
Alveolar CO_2	P_ACO_2

Flows
Air flow	$\dot{V}$
Blood flow	$\dot{Q}$
Inspiratory air flow	$\dot{V}_I$
Expiratory air flow	$\dot{V}_E$
Dead space ventilation	$\dot{V}_D$
Alveolar ventilation	$\dot{V}_A$
Ventilation/perfusion ratio	$\dot{V}/\dot{Q}$

Vascular Pressures
Pulmonary artery	PAP
Pulmonary vein	PVP

Vascular Resistances
Pulmonary	PVR
Systemic	SVR

Fractional Concentrations
Inspired	F_I
Expired	F_E
Alveolar	F_A

Oxygen & Carbon Dioxide Rates
O_2 consumption	$\dot{V}O_2$
Max O_2 consump.	$\dot{V}O_2$ max
CO_2 production	$\dot{V}CO_2$
Resp. exchange ratio	R

Alveolar-Arterial Partial Pressure Differences
Oxygen	A-a PO_2
Carbon dioxide	A-a PCO_2

Central Control
Dorsal respiratory group	DRG
Ventral respiratory group	VRG
Nucleus tractus solitarius	NTS

Diseases
Chronic obstructive pulmonary disease	COPD
Acute/adult respiratory distress syndrome	ARDS
Infant respiratory distress syndrome	IRDS

Pulmonary Function Tests (PFT)
Forced vital capacity	FVC
Forced expiratory volume in 1.0 sec	FEV_1
FEV_1/FVC	FEV%
Forced expiratory flow rate averaged from 25-75% of FVC	$FEV_{25\%-75\%}$
Airway resistance	R_{AW}
Maximum inspiratory pressure	MIP
Maximum expiratory pressure	MEP
Peak expiratory flow rate	PEF (PEFR)
Forced expiratory time	FET
Slow vital capacity	SVC
Closing capacity	CC

Definitions of Pressure Differences	
Transairway	$P_{TA} = P_A - P_{AO}$
Transpulmonary	$P_{TP} = P_{AO} - P_{PL}$
Translung	$P_L = P_A - P_{PL}$
Transthoracic	$P_W = P_{PL} - P_{BS}$
Transrespiratory	$P_{RS} = P_A - P_{BS}$

Index

www.ingramcontent.com/pod-product-compliance
Lightning Source LLC
Chambersburg PA
CBHW041715210326
41598CB00007B/667

9780974165332